WHERE THEY NEED ME

WHERE THEY NEED ME

Local Clinicians and the Workings of Global Health in Haiti

Pierre Minn

CORNELL UNIVERSITY PRESS   ITHACA AND LONDON

First published 2022 by Cornell University Press

Library of Congress Cataloging-in-Publication Data
Names: Minn, Pierre, author.
Title: Where they need me : local clinicians and the workings of global health in Haiti / Pierre Minn.
Description: Ithaca [New York] : Cornell University Press, 2022. | Includes bibliographical references and index.
Identifiers: LCCN 2021058100 (print) | LCCN 2021058101 (ebook) | ISBN 9781501763847 (hardcover) | ISBN 9781501763854 (paperback) | ISBN 9781501763861 (pdf) | ISBN 9781501763878 (epub)
Subjects: LCSH: Medical care—Haiti. | Medical personnel—Haiti. | Medical assistance—Haiti. | Transcultural medical care—Haiti.
Classification: LCC RA456.H3 M56 2022 (print) | LCC RA456.H3 (ebook) | DDC 362.1097294—dc23/eng/20211201
LC record available at https://lccn.loc.gov/2021058100
LC ebook record available at https://lccn.loc.gov/2021058101

To the memories of Anne-Rose "Rosie" Joseph Toussaint (1939–2019) and Rose-Marie Cassagnol Chierici (1942–2020), two extraordinary Haitian women who never doubted that their compatriots deserved better lives, and who inspired thousands to make this goal a reality.

Contents

Acknowledgments

Expressions of gratitude can have many effects. Preparing these acknowledgments made me aware of how many people have helped me over the many years it took to research and write this book. I am reminded of unpaid debts, of obligations that remain unfulfilled, and people who have passed away before seeing this work come to completion. I am also aware that in thanking the individuals below, I expose my networks, affinities, and alliances. I am anxious about leaving someone out, of forgetting kindnesses I might not have deserved in the first place, but received anyway.

In Cap-Haïtien and throughout Haiti, I have had the good fortune of being hosted by an extraordinary community of individuals, the Pères de Sainte-Croix. In particular, Fathers Bernard Antoine, Donald Chéry, Michel Eugène, Pierre-Antoine Mésidor, Pierre Piquion and Frère Jean-Claude Fréchette always made me feel like I had a home and *moun pa*. Friends and mentors in Haiti correct my missteps and give me reasons to want to return: thanks to Patrick Bernard, Jhon Picard Byron, Nanoune Célestin, Mireille Delice, Jean Emmanuel, Eddyles Jacynthe, Shnilove Jean-Louis, Virginie Louis, Nadine Mondestin, Jean-Eddy Rémy, Jean-Eugène Rémy, Pamphile Jean-Pierre Richard, Youseline Telemaque, Thony Voltaire, and the extraordinary staff of the Lambi Fund.

The directors and staff of the Hôpital Universitaire Justinien not only put up with my presence and questions, but they also encouraged me to come back and warned me not to disappear. Dr. Jean-Gracia Coq facilitated my presence at the hospital, from the first day I met him, in a spirit of openness and demonstrating his commitment to fostering research in the institution. Dr. Jean-Géto Dubé continues to make time to meet with me despite his busy schedule and suggests projects for me to work on. The hospital's nurses, pharmacists, support staff, and, in particular, its generations of medical residents have taught me so much about what it means to provide care and healing under difficult circumstances. Dr. Ernst Jasmin at the Département sanitaire du Nord (the northern branch of the Haitian Ministry of Health and Population) has been supportive of my work over the past two decades.

The staff and volunteers of Konbit Sante could not have been more generous and welcoming. In particular, I wish to thank Ruddy Adeca, Fenel Coulanges, Isemanie Georges, Steve and Polly Larned, Eva Lathrop, Tezita Negussie, Nate

Nickerson, and Michael and Wendy Taylor for inviting me to be part of their reflections.

I would also like to gratefully acknowledge the other establishments and organizations that allowed me to learn about their work, including the Hôpital Sacré-Coeur in Milot, Meds and Food for Kids, Alyans Sante Bòy, Haiti Village Health, and CENTRECH.

Portions of this research were presented at Princeton University's Woodrow Wilson School for International Studies, the Yale Center for International and Area Studies, the Moral Economies working group at the University of North Carolina at Chapel Hill, the Department of Anthropology at the University of Wisconsin-Milwaukee, and the Faculté d'ethnologie at the Université d'État d'Haïti.

Funding for this research was provided by the Wenner-Gren Foundation for Anthropological Research, the National Science Foundation, the Social Sciences and Humanities Research Council of Canada, the Fonds de recherche en société et culture du Québec, and the Irmgard Coninx Foundation.

A version of Chapter 4 was published in 2016 as "Components of a Moral Economy: Interest, Credit, and Debt in Haiti's Transnational Healthcare System" in the journal *American Anthropologist* 118 (1): 78–90. Copyright © 2016 by the American Anthropological Association. All rights reserved.

I am grateful to the editorial team at Cornell University Press, in particular Jim Lance, Clare Jones, and Mary Kate Murphy, for their help in bringing this book to fruition.

My introduction to Haiti came while I was working as a research assistant for Nina Glick-Schiller and Georges Fouron, who shared their passion for the country and showed me the importance of Haiti and its diasporas as transnational spaces, and I will be forever grateful to have first traveled to Haiti with Rose-Marie Cassagnol Chierici, an extraordinary anthropologist, teacher, and solidarity activist who, in response to my questions about how I could "make a difference" in the town of Borgne, told me that I should learn Haitian Creole, spend time with farmers, fishermen, market women, and children, in short, learn about and from people before trying to intervene in their lives. Catherine Maternowska pushed me to think about power, inequalities, and justice. Her work remains a model for the type of anthropology that can make the world a better place.

I have had the good fortune of meeting extraordinary mentors during my studies. Linda-Anne Rebhun introduced me to medical anthropology. At McGill University, the Departments of Anthropology and Social Studies of Medicine provided a stimulating academic home. Allan Young was a thoughtful and patient supervisor, who always seemed to know what I was looking for before I did. Sandra Hyde, Margaret Lock, Vinh-Kim Nguyen, and Lisa Stevenson continue to influence my thinking on persons, bodies, health, and medicine. During my postdoctoral fellowship at the University of California, San Francisco, and the University of California, Berkeley, Vincanne Adams, Lawrence Cohen, Sharon Kaufman, and Akhil Mehra offered their generous support and encouragement.

I am grateful to colleagues and students in the Department of Anthropology at the Université de Montréal. I could not ask for a more collegial environment. The Haitian Studies Association (in both its formal and rebellious iterations) has been an exciting intellectual community since I first began traveling to Haiti. Patrick Bellegarde-Smith, Legrace Benson, Jacqueline Épingle, Elizabeth McAlister, and Claudine Michel have provided invaluable guidance and encouragement.

Friends, colleagues, and mentors in medical anthropology and in Haitian studies have provided feedback on this project and support over the years: Greg Beckett, Dörte Bemme, Cal Biruk, Betsey Brada, Paul Brodwin, Sarah Brownell, Manoucheka Celeste, Kyrah Malika Daniels, Pierre-Marie David, Emilio Dirlikov, Vincent Duclos, Toni Eyssallenne, Hannah Gilbert, Gabriel Girard, Annie Jaimes, Hanna Kienzler, Chelsey Kivland, Nolan Kline, Loes Knaapen, Jean-Michel Landry, Peter Locke, Nadève Ménard, Karine Peschard, Raphaëlle Rabanes, Peter Redfield, Jamie Rhoads, Laura Risk, China Scherz, Lynn Selby, Bo-Kyeong Seo, Kathy Smith, Noelle Sullivan, Noémi Tousignant, Grete Viddal, Frantz Voltaire, Claire Wendland, the members of the Q3S writing group, and the late Sam Dubal.

Beth and Chris Daulton, Ashley Diener, Ben Labreche, Andrea Lowgren, Jennifer Malarek, Marie-Paule Préfontaine, Isabelle Saint-Guily, Chantal Smith, Monique Ste-Marie, and John, Mel, and Dale VanderSluis have been pillars of my communities in Montreal and in California.

My late father, Kyungtak Minn, made certain that every door was open to me. My mother Patricia Minn has been a source of unconditional love and support, and a model for how to treat others with care and respect. I am grateful to always be able to count on my sisters Isabelle and Alexandra Minn.

Finally, to my family—Mathieu, Louna, and Ben—thank you for making me feel needed in the best ways possible.

Abbreviations

CARE	Cooperative for Assistance and Relief Everywhere
CIA	Central Intelligence Agency (US)
CIDA	Canadian International Development Agency
FAO	Food and Agriculture Organization of the United Nations
FCO	Foreign and Commonwealth Office (UK)
HAS	Hôpital Albert Schweitzer
HUJ	Hôpital Universitaire Justinien (Cap-Haïtien)
IMF	International Monetary Fund
MINUJUSTH	United Nations Mission for Justice Support in Haiti
MINUSTAH	United Nations Mission for the Stabilization of Haiti
MPCE	Le Ministère de la Planification et de la Coopération Externe (Ministry of Planning and External Cooperation, Haiti)
MSPP	Le Ministère de la Santé Publique et de la Population (Ministry of Public Health and Population, Haiti)
NGO	nongovernmental organization
OAS	Organization of American States
OCHA	Office for the Coordination of Humanitarian Affairs (United Nations)
Oxfam	global organization working to end the injustice of poverty
PAHO	Pan American Health Organization
PARC	Projet d'appui au renforcement des capacités en gestion de la santé en Haïti, Unité de Santé Internationale, Université de Montréal
PEPFAR	President's Emergency Plan for AIDS Relief (US)
PIH	Partners in Health (New England-based organization working in Haiti)
UN	United Nations
UNESCO	United Nations Educational, Scientific, and Cultural Organization
UNHCR	United Nations High Commissioner for Refugees
UNICEF	United Nations Children's Fund
USAID	United States Agency for International Development
USMLE	United States Medical Licensing Examination
WHO	World Health Organization
ZL	Zanmi Lasante (Haitian "sister organization" to Partners in Health)

INTRODUCTION

Dr. Célestin is a small man with freckles and large glasses.[1] He is known among the surgery residents at the Hôpital Universitaire Justinien for being one of the brightest and most talented among them. He has an excellent memory, the ability to pick up new surgical techniques after seeing them performed only once, and the capacity to remain composed even when the lights or air-conditioning in the operating room stop working. I think of him as a quiet person, but know that he has a sense of humor that is both wry and irreverent. Today Dr. Célestin looks tired. We sit on the narrow balcony of the residents' dormitory on dented metal folding chairs, talking about the end of his residency, which is only three months away. He tells me that he will start by looking for work in a hospital run by an international nongovernmental organization (NGO). The pay is better than in Haiti's public hospitals, he says, and doctors and nurses have access to the medicine and materials they need. At the Justinien, like in other government hospitals, surgeries might be canceled simply because there are no sterile drapes or disinfectant. He has had to conduct procedures by the light of his cell phone, and knows that some of his patients may eventually die from preventable infections simply because they cannot afford antibiotics after their operations. Besides, he tells me, doctors in the public system are only paid 300 USD a month. His salary as a full-time medical resident is 200 USD a month, and he has not been paid in seven months.

Like all the other medical residents, Dr. Célestin is worried about his financial situation. His parents, siblings, and extended family are counting on his limited revenue to help cover their basic needs, including housing, school fees, and health care. While working for an NGO is a short-term solution, his ultimate goal is to leave Haiti. "I had a classmate from medical school who got into a residency program in New York," he tells me, "and she's making $90,000 a year! I'm sure she's sending a lot of money back to her family here." He goes on to say, "I wish I could stay in my country to help out in my own way, but I don't know what the country's leaders are going to do. Even if you really want to stay, they'll find a way to discourage you. If that happens, I don't know where I'll end up—in Europe, Canada, or the United States, I don't know . . . a place where they need me."

How is it that a brilliant young physician living in a country with some of the worst health indicators on the planet feels that the places which "need" him are elsewhere? What happens when nurses, doctors, and students from those wealthy and powerful places come to Haiti to provide health services alongside (or in place of) their Haitian counterparts? In countries all over the world where health systems are defined as "weak," where millions of people suffer and die from preventable causes, and where "brain drain" has led to thousands of young, talented clinicians migrating toward the countries that colonized and continue to oppress their nations of origin, these questions force us to confront larger, existential issues: What roles should healers play in their communities? What obligations do people have toward one another in a global context of marked inequalities? In making decisions about what constitutes a good life, what should people strive for?

These questions would become even more pressing for Haitian health workers a few months after I spoke with Dr. Célestin. On January 12, 2010, a 7.0 magnitude earthquake struck the southern part of the Caribbean country, killing tens (possibly hundreds) of thousands, injuring many more, and destroying countless homes, schools, businesses, and government buildings. In October of the same year, a cholera epidemic broke out near a United Nations military base in the center of the country and quickly spread throughout the population. The disease would go on to infect over eight hundred thousand people and kill at least ten thousand individuals, primarily infants and the elderly. Depictions of Haiti in international media have long been negative, but the visual repertoire that followed the earthquake and cholera epidemic was particularly horrifying. Images of bodies stacked like firewood, victims trapped under rubble, and patients dying of diarrhea in crowded cholera treatment centers conveyed scenes of endless need and unbearable suffering. They also suggested that resources, whether financial or human, were absent or insufficient. The events of 2010 and their aftermath prompted an enormous international response: foreign governments pledged billions of dollars; individuals sent donations through text messaging services; and thousands of consultants, employees, and volunteers traveled to

Haiti to provide health and relief services. They quickly got to work creating temporary hospitals, distributing medicines in camps, and setting up new NGOs that would add to the thousands of organizations already active in the country. But it never seemed to be enough.

The discourse of disaster, catastrophe, and emergency that dominated North American media coverage of the earthquake and cholera epidemic eclipsed long-standing and systemic problems: plagued by limited infrastructure, deficient resources, and a lack of political will on the part of national and international actors, health services in Haiti have never come close to meeting the needs of its population. International medical aid in various forms has been streaming into the country for as long as Haitian clinicians have been leaving it, often headed to the very countries that send aid. The quantitative indicators that are most often used to describe the health of a country's population and compare it with those of other nations paint a dismal portrait for Haiti.

Similarly, the numbers that describe Haiti's health system are dire. A 2007 census of Haitian health workers found that there were only .59 nurses and physicians per 1,000 individuals, one of the lowest rates in the world. The World Health Organization (WHO) estimates that it takes a rate of 2.5 health professionals per 1,000 individuals to provide a population with the most basic health services (Dubois, Brunelle, and Rousseau, 2007, 115). In 2017 public spending on health care per capita in Haiti was 13 USD a year (as compared to 180 USD a year in the Dominican Republic and 781 USD in Cuba [World Bank 2017]). While popular forms of healing based on spiritual- and plant-based remedies provide comfort and can heal some basic ailments or treat their symptoms, they are not able to cure or adequately manage the pathologies that are responsible for most deaths in Haiti today: infections, diarrheal diseases,

TABLE 1 Comparison of health indicators in Haiti, neighboring countries, and major aid-donating countries

	HAITI	DOMINICAN REPUBLIC	CUBA	USA	CANADA	FRANCE
Average life expectancy in years (men and women combined)	63.5	73.9	79.1	79.3	82.2	82.4
Maternal mortality (per 100,000 live births)	359	92	39	14	7	8
Infant (0–12 months) mortality rate (per 1,000 live births)	48.22	23.45	3.81	5.56	4.25	3.77
HIV prevalence (%)	2.1	1	.4	.34	.21	.4

Sources: World Health Organization (http://www.who.int/gho/countries/en/); World Factbook (https://www.cia.gov/library/publications/the-world-factbook/rankorder/2155rank.html); CATIE (http://www.catie.ca/en/fact-sheets/epidemiology/epidemiology-hiv-canada).

death during childbirth, and a growing number of chronic illnesses such as diabetes and hypertension (Institut Haïtien de l'Enfance and ICF 2018). Treatments for all of these conditions are considered to be basic care in wealthy countries. Poor economic conditions and deficient biomedical services have combined to make life for many Haitians a daily struggle against disease and an early death.

While the earthquake and cholera epidemic brought increased attention to health conditions in Haiti and attracted new waves of foreign clinicians and medical volunteers, the country was already host to thousands of initiatives sponsored by foreign governments and organizations. Much has been made of Haiti's designation as a "Republic of NGOs" and of the omnipresence of international influences in Haiti's health care system, even though these resources remain incapable of providing sufficient care to the country's population. Little is known, however, about the everyday processes that lead to, shape, and result from medical aid initiatives, and, in particular, the place of Haitian health workers in these programs. Images of medical aid in Haiti generally depict foreign clinicians and Haitian patients, although Haitian nurses, doctors, pharmacists, administrators, and other professionals are increasingly hired to implement aid initiatives and provide services when the *blans* (foreigners) are absent. Haitian orderlies and maintenance staff clean hospitals funded and operated by international groups and governments, while Haitian medical and nursing students study textbooks that have been donated through international educational partnerships. Across the Haitian-Dominican border, the Caribbean Sea, and the Atlantic Ocean, Haitian health workers hope to find employment in Dominican, American, Canadian, or French health institutions. They join the 85 percent of Haitian university graduates who depart from their country, leaving behind crowded clinics and overworked colleagues. The first hospital I visited in Haiti had a single doctor, two nurses, and two nurses' aides. They were the only biomedical professionals for a population of over eighty thousand people, some of whom had to walk eight hours to reach the hospital. Today, that hospital has been transformed through international medical initiatives. Its medical director was trained in Cuba through a Haitian-Cuban medical diplomacy program, and a small American NGO led by a Haitian American university professor funds the hospital in partnership with the Haitian government. The hospital now has a staff of over 130 individuals, including physicians, nurses, dentists, laboratory technicians, pharmacists, administrators, and community health agents.

In this book, I analyze international medical aid in Haiti with an emphasis on the perspectives and experiences of Haitian clinicians, and examine the factors that make emigration appear to be the only viable option to so many of these clinicians. Rather than consider international medical aid and "brain drain" as discrete phenomena, I aim to show how they are in fact two sides of the same coin: the same living and working conditions that drive Haitians to leave their country are those that draw foreign clinicians—mainly from North America and Europe—to Haiti in search of global health "opportunities." This book, therefore, is an anthropological study of transnational health processes. While there are certain categories of individuals that feature prominently in this analysis (namely, young Haitian physicians and North American aid workers and volunteers), and most of my research was conducted in northern Haiti, my goal is not to provide a single or authoritative description of a specific group or institution, but rather to use the tools of ethnography to elucidate how obligations, gift relations, and humanitarianism play out in the Haitian medical context.

Along with a number of anthropologist colleagues, I have chosen to highlight the place of local clinicians in global health interventions (Wendland 2010; Crane 2013; Redfield 2013; Street 2014; McKay 2018; Carruth 2021). In understanding the roles these professionals play in humanitarian interventions and analyzing how they respond to pressures from both impoverished patients and wealthy donors, we learn not only about the workings of contemporary global health programs but also about how individuals negotiate across pronounced resource disparities and cultural divides to work toward better lives for themselves and for those they care for.

Efficacy and Exposé

In writing this account of transnational aid in Haiti, I have attempted to avoid the two genres that are most often used when writing about the topic: evaluations that aim to measure the efficacy of aid interventions and exposés that highlight their failure. The former are generally carried out or commissioned by the agencies or organizations whose interventions are being evaluated with the goal of justifying the use of disbursed resources or to support requests for additional funds. These evaluations tend to involve quantitative measures: accounting of revenues and expenditures, enumerations of activities, inventories of intended versus achieved goals, and indices of changes before or after the intervention. Impacts on the health sector are notoriously difficult to evaluate, given that few health indicators (particularly on a population level), can be directly tied to a specific, discrete intervention. In a recent volume on global health metrics,

Adams (2016) and colleagues show how the quantitative metrics used to evaluate the success of global health interventions focus on increasingly specific and limited indicators while stripping away the context and nuance that are essential for understanding processes and outcomes. Given that these evaluations are often conducted or sponsored by the very organizations whose interventions are being evaluated, the incentives to report successes and positive outcomes are obvious.

In another vein, exposé accounts of international aid have gained visibility in their efforts to critique international interventions for their inefficacy or their role in worsening conditions for the targeted populations. Examples of this genre abound in the popular media: titles such as "International Aid's Dirty Secret" (Ramachandran and Walz 2013), or "The Truth About Foreign Aid" (Sontag 2012) are commonplace in major newspapers. Book-length exposés by journalists, former aid workers, and social scientists have gained prominence in university settings and in the larger public sphere over the past four decades. These include Graham Hancock's *The Lords of Poverty* (1994), David Rieff's *A Bed for the Night* (2002), *Dead Aid* by Dambisa Moyo (2009), and *The White Man's Burden*, by William Easterly (2006). These works draw from both individual case studies and broader economic and demographic data to argue that aid is ineffectual at best and detrimental at worst. They vary in their characterizations of the "true" nature of international aid (an insignificant "Band-Aid" solution, a poorly managed waste of resources, a smokescreen to distract from extractive and neocolonial processes, or a nefarious scheme to keep impoverished populations subjugated). The solutions proposed vary from gradual reforms to the cessation or abolition of aid programs.

Exposés of aid, like all counternarratives, can serve important functions. They call into question powerful structures, amplify critical perspectives that would not reach broader audiences, and have the potential to create needed reforms and decrease harm and injustice. In the case of international aid, a dominant narrative is one in which the citizens, organizations, and governments of wealthy countries are improving the living conditions of populations of poorer countries by helping them meet their basic needs or by facilitating their progress on the road to economic development. Exposé accounts can help us understand why so many international aid initiatives have failed to achieve their stated goals, and why so many of the societies that receive aid remain poor. Descriptions of aid failures or abuse in Haiti have highlighted gross inefficiencies and racism within the American Red Cross (NPR 2015), and revealed instances of sexual misconduct by Oxfam employees (O'Neill 2018). Less dramatic reports include investigations of how aid money was used (including the finding that a significant portion of promised funds were never disbursed or that most funding was channeled to international agencies and organizations rather than to Haitian institutions) or reports of ongoing suffering and poverty in Haiti despite the influx of aid. These investigations, which appear both in the mass media and scholarly studies, generally identify structural and systemic issues as the source of the problem: poor coordination and weak institutions often carry the blame. Moral failures are often hinted at in accusations of graft or corruption (usually leveled at the Haitian government), but these claims are rarely substantiated with specific instances or investigations.

While these exposés are crucial for highlighting the limitations and harmful dimensions of aid, I have made a conscious effort to work outside this genre, or at least not limit myself to it. There are several reasons for this decision. In talking with people in Haiti about aid initiatives, I noticed that, while people were extremely critical of aid in general, they tended to speak positively about specific initiatives that they felt were improving conditions in their communities, and expressed the desire that these initiatives would grow and multiply. Denunciations, while capturing Haitians' frustrations with the inefficacies and harms of aid, are unable to account for the possibility of interventions that have achieved their intended outcomes and have been appreciated by beneficiaries. Approaching a phenomenon as multifaceted as aid in Haiti through the binary categories of success and failure would erase the nuances, textures, and contradictions that characterize any complex process. International aid is extremely diverse in its origins, forms, and outcomes; it mobilizes and affects a wide array of institutions and individuals. Defining what is a successful or a failed intervention is rarely a straightforward process, and the individuals involved in the process may have divergent criteria for what constitutes a desirable outcome. Rather than ask if medical aid in Haiti is *working*, I have chosen to examine the *workings* of aid. This has involved a conscious effort to set aside preexisting assumptions I may have had about my informants' moral qualities and intentions, and allow for the coexistence of failings and triumphs, of mixed motivations and conflicted emotions. It has also meant acknowledging the stakes of my own research and my implications about affective, moral, and economic relationships in Haiti.

This posture has not led to an abandonment of moral claims or commitments my part. Over the years, I have encountered individuals, groups, and initiatives that I feel should not be operating in Haiti (usually because of their limited understanding of the context in which they are working), and others that I have chosen to support with my time, energy, and financial resources. I have also found instances where organizations and individuals I admire greatly have disappointed me, and met others who behave in ways that I find inappropriate but whose work is greatly appreciated by recipient populations, for whom the consequences of international aid can literally be matters of life and death. In this book, I ask readers to take the time to learn about international aid projects and processes in their complexity before weighing in on their moral valence. In an era where information travels rapidly, where images and impressions preclude thicker descriptions and slower assessments, and where there are constant pressures to single out some practices as "best," the impacts of international medical aid and global health projects are too high not to be examined carefully and critically. The choice of a relatively restrained site for this study—northern Haiti—also reflects my commitment to understanding the particularities of aid in a specific time and place, not because what I found there does not exist elsewhere, but if I had been looking at too many places at the same time, I might not have found what I did.

Global Health and Humanitarianism in Haiti

The configuration of resources, institutions, knowledge, and aspirational projects glossed as "global health" emerged in the 1990s at the confluence of several political, economic, and epidemiological factors. As these have been described in detail by a number of anthropologists and historians (Brown, Cueto, and Fee 2006; Lakoff 2010; Crane 2013), I will only mention them summarily here. They include the end of the Cold War and the emergence of the United States as a dominant political and economic superpower; the increased role of nonstate actors (specifically NGOs) in transnational health initiatives; the appearance of the HIV epidemic and the subsequent development of antiretroviral drugs; and advances in information and communication technologies. While its roots in international health and tropical medicine are evident, proponents of global health tend to emphasize its novelty and distinguishing features in light of the paradigms that preceded it (Koplan et al. 2009). Defining what global health is or is not has proven to be a difficult endeavor, in part because its proponents stress its interdisciplinary and inclusive nature. Using more critical perspectives, anthropologists have attempted to describe the unspoken assumptions and logics that shape global health. Lakoff (2010) has identified two "regimes" of global health: global health security and humanitarian biomedicine. The latter has particular relevance for this book:

> Humanitarian biomedicine, in contrast, targets diseases that currently afflict the poorer nations of the world, such as malaria, tuberculosis, and HIV/AIDS. Its problematic is one of alleviating the suffering of individuals, regardless of national boundaries or social groupings. Such intervention is seen as necessary where public health infrastructure at the nation-state level is in poor condition or nonexistent. Humanitarian

biomedicine tends to develop "apolitical" linkages—between nongovernmental organizations, activists, scientific researchers, and local health workers. Its target of intervention is not a collectivity conceived as a national population but rather individual human lives. (60)

Adams (2016) describes global health as "both a response to exigencies of finance, data, and outcomes that have defined the postwar world of international health and a utopian proposition to escape, if not transcend, the problems and perceived lack of success of these arrangements and exigencies" (2). In this and other definitions, we see that global health can refer to the current state of health of the world's population; to an aspirational state in which all people are in good health; and to the programs, strategies, and resources required to move from the former to the latter.

As several authors have noted, Africa has a central place in global health, both as a site where a significant number of projects and resources are directed—particularly those addressing the HIV/AIDS epidemic—and as a site of imagined needs and suffering more broadly (Fourie 2015; A. Patterson 2018). Far from the African continent, Haiti is both marginal and central to global health. Because of the high percentage of Haitians with African ancestry, the country is sometimes represented as being inherently African, although others have shown how Haiti is inarguably a central node in the creation of the New World (Trouillot 1995; Fisher 2004). In her article on global health encounters at a hospital in Botswana, Betsey Brada (2010) illustrates how US medical students come to think of global health as "not here," but elsewhere. From a North American perspective, Haiti is very much "here": in the Eastern Standard Time Zone; a ninety-minute flight from Florida; a site of ongoing US military, economic, and political interventions; and a destination for hundreds of thousands of migrants to the United States and Canada over the past five decades. If remoteness is what makes global health global from a US perspective, Haiti is too close, too American to qualify.

On another level, however, Haiti is a global health case study par excellence. For all that it is lacks in remoteness, representations of Haiti consistently portray a country in desperate need of foreign intervention: poverty (the Haitian poet Jean-Claude Martineau has wryly commented that his nation is the only country to have a last name: "Haiti, the poorest country in the Western Hemisphere"), political instability, high rates of infectious disease, and preventable deaths. Haiti is also the primary point of intervention and analysis of one of the most prominent figures in global health, Dr. Paul Farmer, an American physician and anthropologist who began working in Haiti in the 1980s and cofounded the NGO Partners in Health. Farmer was working in Haiti's impoverished Central Plateau in the years when the first cases of HIV became visible in Haiti. He is best known for his successful initiatives to provide antiretroviral treatments in rural Haiti at a time when few thought this could be logistically or financially possible. Farmer's writings on Haiti, the success of Tracy Kidder's 2003 biography *Mountains beyond Mountains: The Quest of Dr. Paul Farmer, a Man Who Would Cure the World* and the prominence of Partners in Health's activities over the last thirty years have all contributed to Haiti's visibility as a place where global health happens. Farmer died suddenly in his sleep on February 22, 2022, at the age of sixty-two. Ironically, his lifespan fell just short of the average life expectancy in Haiti, the country he often referred to as his "greatest teacher." His influence on health services in Haiti and on global health more broadly cannot be understated.

It should be noted that the Haitian clinicians I worked with rarely referred to their work or the work of their foreign partners as *global health* (or *santé mondiale*) unless these terms were explicit in the programs and institutions they worked with. (*Santé publique, santé communautaire,* or *santé de la population* were much more commonly used to describe interventions that targeted the health of impoverished Haitians, while *aide internationale* or *coopération internationale* referred to internationally funded or operated projects.) However, this may change as a growing number of programs and initiatives using the term *global health* intervene in the country.

Around the same time that global health was emerging as a dominant framework for conceptualizing and combating disease and suffering around the world, a growing number of anthropologists began turning their attention to humanitarianism as an object of study. The anthropology of humanitarianism emerged from several intellectual traditions: studies of international development, a growing interest in refugees and displacement, critical medical anthropology, and a sustained interest in questions related to gift giving, sovereignty, power, and the body (Minn 2007; Ticktin 2014). Rather than coalescing into a single intellectual project, anthropological approaches to humanitarianism have remained diverse, highlighting the inseparability of humanitarian activities from other types of intervention, whether they be evangelical, military, or economic.

Both global health and humanitarianism are prone to being characterized in dichotomies: wealthy vs. poor nations, North vs. South, rich vs. poor, donor vs. recipient. While these binaries do reflect some of the forces at play in transnational medical interventions, the picture they paint grossly oversimplifies the blurred and shifting configurations of institutions, individuals, resources, and discourses in global health and humanitarian projects. Haitian doctors and nurses, like their counterparts in impoverished countries around the world, cannot be easily categorized as donors or recipients, or as wealthy or poor. They occupy a privileged place in their home societies, but generally have access to significantly fewer opportunities than their North American and European colleagues. They are expected to act as impartial intermediaries in distributing foreign resources, but must also respond to the demands of their own kin networks.

While the processes described in this book span several countries and continents, the specific encounters and stories I recount are mostly set in Haiti, specifically in the city of Cap-Haïtien, the country's second largest urban center. Chapter 1 presents the paradox of coordination: while all the actors involved in health interventions in Haiti insist that increased and improved coordination in this sector would be beneficial, they also concur that such coordination is sorely lacking. After detailing some of the structural factors that impede coordination, I go on to explain the strategies used by both Haitians and foreigners to maintain discretion between donors and to keep interventions covert. In Chapter 2, I analyze the work of a small, secular American aid organization whose leaders made an explicit choice not to provide direct clinical services to patients, but rather to work with and through Haitian intermediaries. Their approach provides an opportunity to examine the tensions that exist between tangible and intangible interventions in global health programs. Chapter 3 focuses on the experiences and perspectives of Haitian health professionals in the context of international medical aid and global health. It links their experiences of practicing medicine in a context of pervasive foreign interventions to their projects for migration abroad, primarily to aid-sending countries. In the following chapter, I describe a moral economy of international medical aid in Haiti, and examine the morally saturated categories of interest, credit, and debt in order to reveal some of the less visible dimensions of aid encounters. The fifth and final chapter presents an analysis of three archetypal figures that emerge in portrayals of aid interventions in Haiti: saints, villains, and champions. I use the case of Paul Farmer to examine how and why foreign health professionals (particularly physicians) are depicted as saints, while Haitian clinicians are often cast as champions or villains—either self-sacrificing for a cause exterior to themselves or morally corrupt and a threat to the integrity of humanitarian endeavors.

Methodology and Fieldwork

I conducted the core of the ethnographic research for this book during fourteen months of fieldwork in Haiti between the fall of 2007 and the spring of 2009. Prior to this period, I had spent approximately one year in rural areas of northern and northeastern Haiti conducting research on health conditions and medical services. I selected the city of Cap-Haïtien as my primary field site in part because of my familiarity with the area and my existing network of local contacts, but mostly because I wanted to examine international medical aid in a densely populated urban setting outside of the capital of Port-au-Prince, where nearly all urban ethnographies of Haiti have been conducted (see, for example, Maternowska 2006; Giafferi-Dombre 2007; James 2010; Beckett 2019; Kivland 2020). Working in Cap-Haïtien allowed me to observe the challenges faced by large health institutions outside of the capital in the context of a highly centralized health system.

The bulk of my research took place at the Hôpital Universitaire Justinien (HUJ) in the heart of Cap-Haïtien, Haiti's second largest city. Founded in 1890 by wealthy citizens in order to keep the city's destitute out of public view (Constant 1967), the hospital was administered by an order of French nuns until the early 1990s when it was taken over by the Haitian government. As Alice Street (2014) notes, hospitals in postcolonial settings represent sites for state-building efforts by foreign governments and agencies, but these same efforts produce states that fail to "see, recognize or care for [their] subjects" (22). When I first arrived at the Justinien, the hospital had 240 beds, making it the second largest in the country after l'Hôpital Général in Port-au-Prince. Shortly after I began my research, the Justinien's medical and executive directors wrote a notice stating that I would be at the hospital for a prolonged period of time conducting a study on international interventions and sent copies to all the department heads in the institution. I subsequently saw the notice posted on the walls of the various departments next to other official announcements and flyers. This simple act formally legitimated my presence at the hospital and greatly facilitated my presence in the Justinien's offices and clinical spaces. Because I was often seen in the presence of international aid groups, many people assumed that I was a member of such a group. I did my best to correct this assumption by repeatedly explaining the purpose of my research, increasing my presence at the hospital after foreign teams had departed, and taking small actions to distinguish myself from the foreign teams (such as not arriving at or departing from the hospital with them, visibly paying separately for my meals in hotels or restaurants, and sitting or socializing with Haitians when mixed groups divided along national or linguistic lines). As in any field setting, it was impossible for me to determine others' impressions of my identity or purpose. After a few months, some of the hospital staff I had become friendly with informed me of rumors that I was working for the CIA.[2] In the streets of Cap-Haïtien, I was regularly mistaken for a Catholic priest, a Protestant missionary, a Dominican businessman, or a UN worker. When asked, I stated that I was a Canadian anthropologist doing research on health care and international aid.

Before beginning the research for this book, I was aware of five international bodies providing aid at the Justinien, and assumed that I would encounter about ten in all. Before the 2010 earthquake, I had identified thirty-five governmental and nongovernmental agencies and organizations that were directly and indirectly providing some form of support to the hospital, and more have appeared since I completed my fieldwork. It was apparent even early on during my research that I would be unable to thoroughly investigate all of these sources of aid. Instead, I chose initiatives based on the access I could obtain to informants involved in them, and attempted to select forms of aid that were diverse in their origins, structures, and activities. The aid group I had the most contact with was Konbit Sante, a small American NGO working in multiple areas of the hospital. Other groups I spent significant periods of time with included a team of Dominicans and Americans who traveled to Haiti to provide orthopedic surgeries; an organization of Haitian Canadians that organized workshops for nursing students and provided donations of medical equipment for several of the hospital's departments; an American NGO that provided nutritional therapy to malnourished children; and a Florida university–based family medicine residency program for Haitian medical residents that also oversaw the Justinien's HIV treatment programs. I chose not to investigate certain organizations in depth because of their relatively minor involvement in the hospital (i.e., periodic or one-time donations, etc.). Other agencies worked through the organizations I examined more directly—for example, the US Centers for Disease Control partially funded the Florida-based university's work at the Justinien, but were not otherwise present at the hospital. Some organizations were based in distant locations and difficult to access (such as a group in Germany that funded the ophthalmology department). Access to a medical aid initiative was only explicitly denied in one case, that of the Cuban medical brigades.[3]

When foreign groups were physically present at the hospital, I accompanied them during their activities. This ranged from translating in meetings with the hospital administrators and staff to sitting in on consultations with patients and unloading donated equipment from shipping containers. I also met with the groups at their hotels, joining them for meals and the long discussions that followed their days at the hospital. I conducted formal interviews with two dozen international aid workers and had more informal conversations with many more. When foreign teams were not present, I followed the activities of the hospital's medical staff, in particular those who worked closely with international programs. These included nurses, physicians, administrators, accountants, orderlies, cleaning staff, drivers, and trainees. I became particularly interested in the work and experiences of the hospital's fifty-four medical residents. These recent graduates of Haitian medical schools in Port-au-Prince were undertaking three- to four-year residencies at the Justinien in a variety of medical specialties, including pediatrics, obstetrics-gynecology, internal medicine, surgery, family medicine, and urology. The residents ranged in age from mid-twenties to mid-thirties, and while medicine in Haiti has historically been dominated by men, there were slightly more female than male residents at the hospital. I conducted semistructured interviews with fifty-two of the residents to gain insight into their relationships with and perspectives on international interventions at the hospital. I also interviewed them about other dimensions of their lives related to transnationalism, including their experiences abroad and their future career plans, which in most cases involved emigration. I conducted the interviews in Haitian Creole and in French. Over time, I developed friendships with many of the residents, and had the opportunity to meet their family members, travel with them to their hometowns, and participate in social events such as trips to historic sites, weddings, and graduation ceremonies. I have maintained some of these relationships in the years that followed my initial fieldwork, reconnecting with the former residents in Haiti, Canada, and the United States.

In addition to my research in Cap-Haïtien, I also traveled to rural field sites in northern Haiti to visit private hospitals and clinics and to follow weeklong mobile medical campaigns by visiting foreign teams. These experiences provided contrasting examples and data to the findings from the Justinien, and gave me a better sense of how medical aid operates in diverse forms throughout Haiti. Finally, I conducted research in the American and Canadian cities where selected aid organizations are based, including Portland, Memphis, and Montreal, where I visited organizations' offices, attended meetings and events, and interviewed North American staff and volunteers. The observations and interviews from these locations gave me insights into how international aid workers and volunteers interpret and give meaning to their work in Haiti in very different contexts, and how they translate situations, encounters, and projects from Haiti into narratives and appeals that can reach North American audiences.

Most of the groups I focused my attention on were secular in nature. This is due both to circumstance and to a conscious effort on my part. The majority of international aid groups and organizations active at the Justinien were not religiously affiliated. As an officially secular public institution, the hospital tends to attract partnerships with large multinational agencies, national governments, universities, and civic institutions.[4] Religiously affiliated hospitals and clinics in Haiti are much more likely to receive support from international religious bodies such as individual churches, church networks, or religious NGOs. In addition, I was particularly interested in following the work of secular organizations to examine changes in international medical aid in recent decades. While faith-based aid and development initiatives are extremely active in Haiti and elsewhere

(Bornstein 2005; Hefferan 2007), secular medical aid organizations in the country have increased in prominence in recent years. This is not to claim that the secular groups I studied are not drawing from or influenced by an established Judeo-Christian tradition, or that aid administrators and recipients in Haiti do not interpret their secular donors' actions in religious terms. Rather, I was interested in exploring the distinct logics and values that secular organizations draw from and express in carrying out their activities.

Once it became clear that my primary goal was not to expose their faults or failings, nearly all the groups I approached welcomed my presence. After it became apparent that I would be at the Justinien for a significant period of time, most of them asked if I could assist them in their activities by translating, helping with logistics when they were not in Haiti, and sharing the results of my research so that they could improve their programs. In her research on transnational projects in Mozambique, Ramah McKay (2018) found her interlocutors were already engaged in sophisticated critiques of how humanitarianism and aid work; she contends that a critique is "not only the outside stance of an observer looking on, but [it] also constitutes the object of study" (197). Similarly, many of the organizations I encountered, Konbit Sante in particular, were already involved in a process of critical self-reflection about the impacts of their interventions and regularly asked me for my insights and analyses of their work, even when some of my findings identified errors and shortcomings. The Haitian clinicians, health workers, and administrators I encountered were at times ardent supporters and active critics of international interventions and, for the most part, were eager to share their perspectives and experiences. At times, I had to overcome some initial reticence. Those who work in Haiti's health sector are used to regular comings and goings by foreigners, many of whom arrive with questionnaires and reports to fill out. After seeing me at the hospital for periods of weeks, months, and eventually years, however, my interlocutors came to understand that my engagement with their workplace would be for the long haul. Since I began my research, I have made efforts to share the results of my work in Haiti through individual conversations, mentorship for junior researchers, talks, workshops and training for hospital employees, and appearances on local television and radio stations. This book (and its forthcoming translations for Haitian audiences) represents a continued effort to share my findings and challenge not only assumptions about the workings of aid in Haiti but also the ways in which questions about aid are framed and developed.

THE LOGIC OF UNCOORDINATION

A paradox emerged early on during my conversations about coordination with actors involved in international medical aid in Haiti. When compared with issues such as funding priorities, the efficacy of interventions, or the nature of obligations, nearly all of my interlocutors—whether they were Haitian, foreign, donors, recipients, volunteers, professional aid workers, or simply casual observers—spoke about the problem of coordination in remarkably consistent terms. I heard over and over that the coordination of international medical aid in Haiti is minimal, insufficient, or completely absent, and that this lack produces undesirable effects, such as wasted resources, duplication of services, and, ultimately, the deterioration of the health of Haiti's population. Everyone I spoke with agreed that increased coordination would be beneficial, with many individuals stating that coordination was the single most important factor in improving the process of aid in the country. Similar claims appear regularly in public commentary, notably in the statements of government leaders, policy analysts, and journalists. The voices decrying the lack of coordination and its nefarious effects increased in number and intensity after the January 2010 earthquake.

Herein lies the paradox: If everyone involved in the aid process agrees on the importance of increased coordination, why is it absent? How should we interpret the apparent discrepancy between a unanimously identified objective and its elusive achievement? I propose four possibilities. The first is that my informants and other commentators are speaking disingenuously. That is to say, they are not sincere in their statements that they favor more coordination, but simply say so because of pressures to conform to a popular and widespread opinion.

A position denouncing a lack of coordination resembles a stance taken against corruption, or pollution, or delinquency. I never heard any of my informants say that medical aid in Haiti was sufficiently or excessively coordinated and can imagine that a person expressing such an opinion would face strong rebuttals. However, even if the term is often used in vague or unspecified terms, nearly all of my informants in Haiti had ideas about what *coordination* would entail (for example, that donors and recipients would communicate transparently with each other), and what benefits it would bring (that populations in need would receive the goods and services essential to live healthy lives). They provided specific anecdotes of unfortunate events they attributed to a lack of coordination. I also heard of and witnessed firsthand some efforts to coordinate medical aid initiatives, some of which I will describe later in this chapter. As a result, I believe that when most people who have direct experience with international aid in Haiti complain about a lack of coordination, they are genuine in their claims and base their opinions on empirical examples.

The second possibility is that coordination exists, but it is not identified as such by commentators. I believe this to be partially true, in the sense that much of the coordination I observed during my research—including the sharing of information, collaborations on specific initiatives and projects, and harmonious interactions between diverse actors—was informal and localized; it would not be recognized as coordination on a larger or more formal scale. The issue here may be one of scope. When my informants decried a lack of coordination, their frame of reference was often Haiti on a national level. The same is true in reports by outside analysts and commentators. Many of those calling for increased coordination may not perceive or acknowledge the diverse forms of collaboration and coordination that take place on a small scale or outside of formal institutional frameworks. However, many informants complained about a lack of coordination at the local or regional level as well, citing examples where organizations or agencies operating at a specific site act in ways that appear uncoordinated.

The third possibility is that coordination of international medical aid in Haiti is simply impossible, due to the scope of the actors involved and the scale of their areas of intervention or because of the actors' own personal limitations and short-comings. In addition to state actors (various branches of the Haitian government, foreign governments, the United Nations and its numerous agencies), the number of NGOs in Haiti is commonly cited as a factor impeding the coordination of aid efforts. While 605 NGOs were registered with the Ministry of Planning and External Cooperation in 2015–16 (Ministère de la Planification et de la Coopération Externe, n.d.), the estimated number of unregistered NGOs operating in the country ranges from 3,000 to 10,000, a significant percent of which conduct some kind of health intervention. (These calculations generally do not account for private clinics or health establishments.) While this scope is daunting, and the coordination of so many diverse actors is difficult to envision, dramatic improvements in telecommunications (primarily through cellular phones) and new internet-based technologies have greatly facilitated the logistical dimensions of communicating and coordinating in Haiti. These technologies remain inaccessible to many people in Haiti, but they have facilitated communication and coordination among key players and stakeholders, and will continue to influence how coordination occurs. Since actors involved in the aid process could often name precise situations where coordination was technically possible but did not occur, technical limitations cannot be identified as the sole cause of a lack of coordination.

The fourth and final explanation for the discrepancy between a call for increased coordination and its persistent absence is the one to which I will devote the greater part of this chapter: the number of compelling incentives for foreigners and Haitians involved in international medical aid *not* to coordinate. Phrased in more positive terms, these individuals and organizations have a variety of reasons to favor autonomy and discretion over coordination. Before turning to these reasons, however, I will briefly detail how those involved in the aid process define coordination and how it appears in institutional discourse. I will also address some of the more immediately apparent factors impeding coordination—namely, time, language, and organizational leadership. These factors are directly related to the specific ethnographic context, but should also be considered as factors impeding the coordination of aid in other settings.

Defining Coordination

Coordination in the aid sector generally implies interventions being planned in ways that account for the existence and actions of multiple actors, whether they be other donors or recipients. In a context where interventions are organized around providing resources that are absent, it is not surprising that Haitian medical staff associated a lack of coordination with the donation of unnecessary or useless items by foreign aid groups and agencies, as well as the duplication, redundancy, and waste of resources. The following statements are typical of the comments made by health care professionals, focusing on the logistics of material donation, the visibility of results, the persistence of problems despite the presence of multiple aid groups, and the incapacity of the Haitian state:

> Here's why coordination is important. International aid groups send us certain kinds of material, but we don't really use them. They could send

us the things we do use; there are a lot of things we're lacking. I think that's a lack of coordination.

If aid were coordinated, that would let you see the results of what you've done.

The problem is duplication. You have multiple NGOs that are intervening in the same area, and the problem still doesn't get solved.

We don't know what we want, and when we start doubting, that makes aid move backwards, because no one knows what we want.

There are a lot of organizations working in the dark, and each person does what he or she wants. The state isn't capable of taking control of the situation, to say, "OK, everyone's under my control. You have to do this, you do that, we have to meet once a week to report on what's not been done."

Haitians outside of the medical sector make similar claims, reflecting a widespread sentiment throughout the country that international aid more broadly is poorly coordinated. At times, critiques from outside medical establishments identify medical workers as responsible for or benefiting from this lack of coordination, such as when hospital employees are accused of pilfering donated supplies for use in their private clinics, or of charging fees for services that have already been subsidized by international bodies.

Foreign informants echoed their Haitian counterparts' complaints about the negative consequences that result from a lack of coordination. Established institutions and organizations often resented the arrival of new groups that periodically came through existing catchment areas to conduct mobile clinics and distribute vitamins, medications, clothing, and other goods. These groups generally do not have access to patients' medical histories and rarely create their own documentation, are often unfamiliar with the pathologies that are frequent in rural Haiti, and do not always make provisions for follow-up care. Among other factors, coordination for many foreign informants involved new or recent aid initiatives gaining awareness of existing services in an area, and working with them, rather than on their own. For those foreigners committed to working with the Haitian state, the existing services also included those offered by state-run public establishments. These individuals were likelier than others to identify the Haitian government as the entity that should be responsible for coordinating all health activities in the country.

While discourse about the importance of aid coordination in Haiti has proliferated among aid organizations, government agencies, and in North American print media since the January 2010 earthquake, it can be traced in its current form to the mid-1990s. Specifically, the end of the US-initiated international embargo on Haiti in 1994 led to the resumption and initiation of diverse international aid initiatives (Interim Cooperation Framework 2006, 5, 44). In 1999 a UN advisory group on Haiti found that

> strengthening the leadership role of the government in aid coordination is key to making Haiti's cooperation with its international development partners more effective. Decades of institutional instability have adversely affected the coordination capacities of the government accumulated in previous years. The situation steadily further worsened following the 1991 military coup when the constitutional government went into exile and the void in development was filled by international donors and NGOs. Since the return of the constitutional government in October 1994, the institutions officially charged with aid coordination have found it increasingly difficult to effectively coordinate the activities of most external partners. This is partly due to donor-driven initiatives and the fact that many of these partners, including some non-governmental organizations have not yet shed the isolated operational practices adopted during the embargo years. (UN Ad Hoc Advisory Group on Haiti 1999)

Responses to the devastating floods in the city of Gonaïves in 2004 also brought the subject of coordination to the fore. Coordination of aid in Haiti has been the primary topic of several international meetings and conferences. A 2007 meeting hosted by the World Bank and the Government of Haiti convened representatives from nine nations, the European Commission, the Organization of American States (OAS), the International Monetary Fund (IMF), the Pan American Health Organization (PAHO), and the UN (World Bank 2007). The purpose of the meeting was to discuss coordination between donors and the Government of Haiti, as well as among donors themselves. In 2009 the Government of Mexico hosted a "Hemispherical Conference on Coordination for International Cooperation with the Republic of Haiti." The same year, the Canadian minister of International Cooperation reported after a trip to Haiti: "I'm proud that Canada is taking leadership on Haiti, especially on improving coordination and coherence among donors to ultimately deliver results. . . . By working together, we can seize upon a unique opportunity to bring hope to this country" (CIDA 2009).[1]

In both institutions' and individuals' discourses on coordination, the achievement of intended results looms large. Conversely, the absence of such results (in this case, the persistence of poor health conditions in the Haitian population) signals a lack of coordination. Ironically, it is this same emphasis on results—immediate, dramatic, and visible—that often leads to uncoordinated activity, as actors move to act quickly and "get the job done." While some obstacles to coordination can be addressed through policy measures, others are related to more structural issues, including the basic issue of language.

Language

Language poses a formidable barrier to the coordination of international interventions in Haiti, despite the country being one of the world's most linguistically homogenous nations. Very few foreign aid workers or volunteers in the country speak or understand Haitian Creole. This is true even among those who have had significant or long-standing involvement with the country. I met a physician who told me that he was on his 104th trip to Haiti, but could not function there without a translator. In Port-au-Prince, I met employees of government aid agencies and large aid organizations who had been living in Haiti for several years uninterrupted and were still unable to introduce themselves in Creole. The short-term volunteers I met often knew simple phrases and expressions, but the only foreigners I met who were able to communicate fluently with Haiti's unilingual Creole majority were those aid workers, missionaries, and researchers who had lived for significant periods (upwards of six months) in the country's rural areas or secondary cities. There are several factors that explain these phenomena. There are relatively few resources for learning Creole outside of Haiti, particularly if one lives in an area without a significant Haitian immigrant population. In addition, Haitian Creole's status as a stigmatized language—one that developed only three centuries ago under colonial slavery, and many of whose speakers today are marginalized, impoverished, and illiterate—plays a role in its lack of uptake by foreigners. A Belgian aid worker confessed to me, "Whenever I speak Creole, I feel like I'm speaking bad French." Many foreigners I met in Haiti were uncertain if Creole was a "real" language, a dialect of French, or "broken French."

For those foreigners who do learn Creole, even this may not be enough to overcome the significant language barriers. While Haitian Creole is the mother tongue of nearly all Haitians (the exception being a small percentage of French/Creole bilinguals among Haiti's middle and elite classes), French remains the language for most official communication in elite spaces, such as schools, government establishments, courts, and health centers. Although estimates of French fluency among Haitians are generally below 15 percent of the population, the language has long been entrenched as a powerful symbol of privilege and social status (Valdman 1984, 77–82). In institutions such as hospitals and government offices, French is commonly used among professional staff. Formal presentations and meetings often begin in French, although speakers routinely switch to Creole when discussions become more animated and heated. While there is a concerted effort to increase the number of Creole texts in the country, most of the printed materials produced in Haiti are in French, and the forms, manuals, and documents that accompany interventions from overseas are generally in English or French. While French and Haitian Creole are related (the former was the principal source of much of the latter's lexicon), they are not mutually intelligible. This has several impacts on transnational encounters. I often met American aid workers who had invested a great deal of energy in becoming fluent in Creole, but who remained unable to participate in interactions in French. These interactions often had high stakes, given that they often took place in sites of decision making and power. Conversely, many Haitian professionals have never learned to read or write Haitian Creole, and feel more comfortable reading and producing documents in French.

For some international aid workers and volunteers, communicating in Creole or French is simply not a priority. An American doctor once told me, "We speak the same language: medicine!" Oftentimes, foreign volunteers are able to communicate with Haitian health professionals in English, as many of the latter (particularly physicians) speak or at least understand English. Contact with patients—who rarely spoke English in the encounters I observed—was particularly challenging, and organizations providing clinical services usually ensured that a translator was present. Nevertheless, language barriers in international interventions are real, particularly for those who are monolingual speakers of subaltern languages. I observed countless cases where, despite the presence and hard work of competent translators, meanings were distorted and intentions misread. At the administrative level, translation can facilitate formal meetings, but it is largely inadequate for the kinds of casual conversations and informal socializing that build collegial and amicable relationships and help lay the foundation for mutual trust and collaboration. Not surprisingly, most of the effort I witnessed to learn another language has been on the part of Haitians, who recognize that proficiency in French, English, and Spanish has numerous economic and social advantages.

Language, therefore, became a major obstacle to coordinating the diverse parties active in medical interventions in Haiti. The four most relevant languages were Creole (spoken by the entirety of the Haitian population and the sole language of a majority of Haitians), French (used in elite spheres in Haiti and the first language of many aid workers and volunteers from France, Quebec, Belgium, and Switzerland), Spanish (used by Cubans and the Haitian graduates of Cuban medical schools, Dominicans, Spaniards, Venezuelans, and other Latin Americans), and English (used by Americans, Anglophone Canadians, aid workers from non-francophone or non-hispanophone countries, and members of the Haitian American diaspora who do not speak Creole or French). Among other factors, the possibility of becoming fluent in a new language depends largely on time, both in terms of time devoted to learning, and the overall duration of the period dedicated to learning and practice. Time in and of itself is also an important factor that influences the coordination of international medical aid in Haiti.

Time

Many of the foreigners involved in interventions in Haiti do not live there full time. This is particularly true in areas such as Cap-Haïtien. While government aid agencies and leaders of large aid groups do have expatriate employees, they tend to live in Port-au-Prince. In other parts of the country, aid groups rely almost exclusively on Haitian staff, and foreign personnel and volunteers typically come to Haiti for short stays.[2] While some of the directors and leaders of medical aid groups spend up to several months of each year in Haiti, many are there for only a few weeks per year. Even those who spend significant time in Haiti often break up these stays into many short trips at regular intervals in order to manage work and family obligations in their home countries. As a result, when these leaders are in Haiti, they usually have an enormous number of tasks to accomplish in relatively brief periods of time. It is not unusual to see group leaders working twenty-hour days in Haiti—filled with tasks that include conducting site visits; filling out paperwork; purchasing supplies; carrying out assessments; and providing guidance to new employees, group members, and volunteers. In addition, leaders may be providing clinical services and other forms of aid to an unending stream of patients and solicitors, whose number always grows as the word spreads that a foreign aid worker is present, especially when the worker is one with access to resources and decision-making power. Finally, the leaders of foreign medical aid groups spend much of their time in Haiti in lengthy meetings.

Various types of meetings are among the most time-consuming activities for aid workers and volunteers, particularly for leaders and other members with authority in the group. These include meetings with local staff and partners to discuss programs and working conditions, discussions with government officials and other authorities, and internal meetings (particularly if teams of aid workers from disparate locations outside of Haiti have come together to work or volunteer). Meetings are both occasions where coordination can take place and time-consuming events that can preclude the possibility of coordination.

Meetings in Haiti are notoriously lengthy. While informal negotiations and quick discussions can take place in hallways and from the windows of passing vehicles, formal meetings often last for many hours. Discussions between speakers of different languages take even longer because of translation (sometimes

between more than two languages) and the need to clarify resulting misunder-
standings or ambiguities. Tardy arrivals often lead to delays and postponements.[3]
Meetings frequently begin with a song and a prayer, particularly if they take place
in rural areas or under the auspices of a religious establishment or organization. This is generally followed by self-introductions by each of the participants.
Detailed agendas are rarely established ahead of time, and some participants may
often have only a very general idea of what will be discussed. I often sat in on
meetings where participants confessed that they did not know why they were
there, but had come simply because they had been told to by a superior.

Once the introductions have been completed, a leader figure typically begins
by announcing the topic of discussion, providing background information, and
raising issues related to the topic. This person is generally the individual who
convened the meeting or a person of high status (oftentimes an older man with
a respected status: physician, government official, religious leader, etc.). Formal
meetings, particularly in urban areas or those that include bilingual participants,
usually begin in French, even in the presence of monolingual Creole speakers. It
is not uncommon, however, for the participants to switch into Creole at a certain
point in the meeting. This move both results from and contributes to more animated discussions, heated exchanges, and direct communication. It also allows
for new configurations in terms of the meeting participants: who is able to follow
and participate in the conversation, and who is excluded.

An important feature of many meetings in Haiti is the expectation that all
participants be allowed to express themselves and comment on a given situation.
This is not to say that preexisting hierarchies, interpersonal tensions, or other factors constraining an individual's capacity to speak in a group setting disappear.
Rather, it became clear during my research that most practices of exclusion took
place before meetings were convened, so that if a person was present at a meeting,
it meant that the organizer or organizers had taken the participant's presence and
potential contributions into account, as well as his or her discretion regarding
any sensitive material that might emerge during the meeting.

These assumptions led to some uncomfortable situations when foreigners organized meetings. In many of the Haitian-organized meetings I attended
during my work, participants tended to be of roughly the same occupational
or social status. Physicians met with other physicians, head nurses with head
nurses, and support staff with support staff. In cases such as the latter, the meeting might be run by a higher-level employee or administrator whose authority set him or her apart from the rest of the group, but the other participants
were relatively homogeneous in terms of their status in the hospital's hierarchy.
Foreigners, however—who were often unaware of the specific status and class
distinctions that might characterize a group in Haiti, or who felt that meetings

between individuals from disparate backgrounds and positions were necessary for the success of their intervention—might bring together a hospital director, a janitor, a medical student, an ambulance driver, and a folk healer for a meeting that would never have taken place under any other circumstance. The outcomes of such meetings varied greatly depending on the personalities of the individuals involved, the topic being discussed, and the context in which the meeting took place. Some degenerated into shouting matches such as those among clinic staff described by Catherine Maternowska (2006, 94–95) while the tone of others remained courteous and collegial.

Talk about meetings, their purpose and effectiveness reflected the ambivalent attitudes both Haitians and non-Haitians had about them. For my Haitian informants, *rankont* or *reyinyon* can be a waste of time—a seemingly endless set of rhetorical exercises that lead to no or insignificant changes in their working conditions. They are particularly critical of *seminè* (seminars or workshops) hosted by international groups because these often take place in expensive hotels and resorts and exemplify the immoral waste of resources in a context of great scarcity. On the other hand, Haitians involved in international medical aid also appreciate meetings where they feel they can air their concerns and come into contact with the individuals responsible for aid projects. Complaints about long, ineffective meetings coexist with frustrations that international donors do not always take the time to listen to Haitians' concerns and ideas, and that there are limited opportunities for communicating grievances or suggestions. Exclusion from meetings is also a cause for disappointment and resentment.

International aid workers and volunteers also express ambivalence about meetings. They frequently complain about their length, and about physical discomforts such as cramped quarters, uncomfortable seats, and high temperatures. Translators often begin to falter several hours into the meeting (often after the discussions have switched into Creole, making the negotiations less intelligible to non-Haitians). The lack of a structured agenda and contradictory input from diverse actors often increases the level of frustration. Yet meetings represent an important point of direct contact with people that most foreigners involved in international aid do not have access to for much of the year. Many have complained to me about the difficulty of getting information from Haiti through phone calls and emails, stating that ambiguous or complex situations are only ever clarified during face-to-face encounters. In addition, for groups that prioritize structural changes in Haiti's health care system rather than the provision of clinical services or material goods, meetings are an opportunity to work toward their goals of increasing communication among diverse or estranged parties, streamlining bureaucratic processes, and consolidating ideas and resources to solve health problems. I heard repeatedly from members of an American NGO that one of their main goals is to "get people talking to each other who wouldn't be talking otherwise." This statement is not limited to meetings between heterogeneous groups like those mentioned earlier. Both international workers and Haitian hospital staff at the Hôpital Universitaire Justinien complained about the lack of regular and routine meetings of the heads of the hospital's various departments. Such meetings tend to only take place in times of acute crisis, such as during the residents' strike or after the 2010 earthquake.

The time constraints that result from many aid workers' relatively brief trips to Haiti and leaders' packed schedules play a role in impeding coordination, at least in the sense that they do not allow for proactive networking and partnership development. International medical aid workers and volunteers who travel to Haiti for short stays generally spend most of their time at their specific intervention sites, and interact primarily with other members of their own group or preexisting partners. New contacts and partnerships often develop out of chance encounters. For example, it is not unusual for members of aid groups to strike up conversations with each other in the waiting room at the small airport in Cap-Haïtien. Because of poor infrastructure in many parts of Haiti (particularly in terms of roads, communication, etc.), it has been common for foreign groups to be working in the same area without communicating, or even being aware of each other's existence. This has changed significantly in recent years with the increased availability of cellular phones in Haiti, as well as the proliferation of internet-based programs and technologies that allow a greater number of groups and individuals to be identified, located, and contacted. Now that communication among the various actors involved in medical aid has become easier, and the tools essential for coordinating have become more numerous and more accessible, older questions of leadership and responsibility have become increasingly relevant.

Leadership

The issue of group structure and leadership is another factor that influences if and how the various actors involved in international health interventions coordinate their efforts. Many of the groups, organizations, and agencies I followed were led by a prominent, charismatic leader. Certain agencies and large NGOs have more diffused leadership and decision-making processes, either because of personalities, bureaucratic structures whose size or density discourage charismatic leadership, or frequent turnover of staff. However, many of the initiatives I observed were spearheaded by a single individual whose activities, resources, and influence were indispensable for the group's operation. This is apparent to the Haitian intermediaries and recipients, who, in addition to referring to a group by its formal name, often use terms such as *ekip Doktè Wilè* (Dr. Wheeler's team) or *gwoup Natali* (Nathalie's group). In some cases, the term *team* or *group* is omitted, making it sound as though the individual is acting in isolation.[4]

What impact does this have on coordination? While the tendency for groups to be led by charismatic leaders facilitates coordination in certain circumstances, it can also impede it and lead to many of the factors my informants complained about: isolation, waste, chaos, and redundancy. Concentrated and charismatic leadership means that when leaders encounter a potential partner, they can often make rapid and unencumbered decisions about what type of relationship they could have with such a partner, what resources and information could be shared, and the general terms of collaboration and partnership. For example, if the head of an organization offering primary health care in a small village meets the leader of an organization providing donations of soap throughout Haiti, the former could single-handedly initiate a partnership that would result in soap being distributed in the village. While most of the organizations I studied are typically governed by administrative boards, these are generally made up of people living outside of Haiti, whose experience in the country is limited and who are often willing to defer judgment about partnerships and programs to the group's executive leader. I observed that a great deal of the collaborative work and partnerships among international aid bodies in Haiti, both formal and informal, are based on individuals' affinities and ties.

The converse reality, however, is that charismatic and concentrated leadership in groups also impedes coordination. As I mentioned earlier, group leaders who do not live in Haiti are generally extremely busy and overextended during their trips to the country, and coordination is not always a priority. If other members of the group, Haitian or foreign, do not have the authority to communicate on the group's behalf or make decisions about the terms of coordination, it may simply not take place. In addition, the prominence of individual leaders in the activities of aid groups allows for the development of intergroup conflicts resulting from clashes in personalities and temperaments. Two groups that might have common or complementary goals, activities, and resources may operate in isolation from each other because their leaders had an altercation or dislike each other's personalities. (The same, of course, holds true for relationships with Haitian institutions, both public and private, many of which have concentrated leadership). In some cases, individualistic attitudes and a desire for personal prominence undermine working with other actors.

The factors I have just detailed—language, time, and leadership—are structural and logistical considerations essential for understanding the presence or absence of coordination of international medical interventions in Haiti.

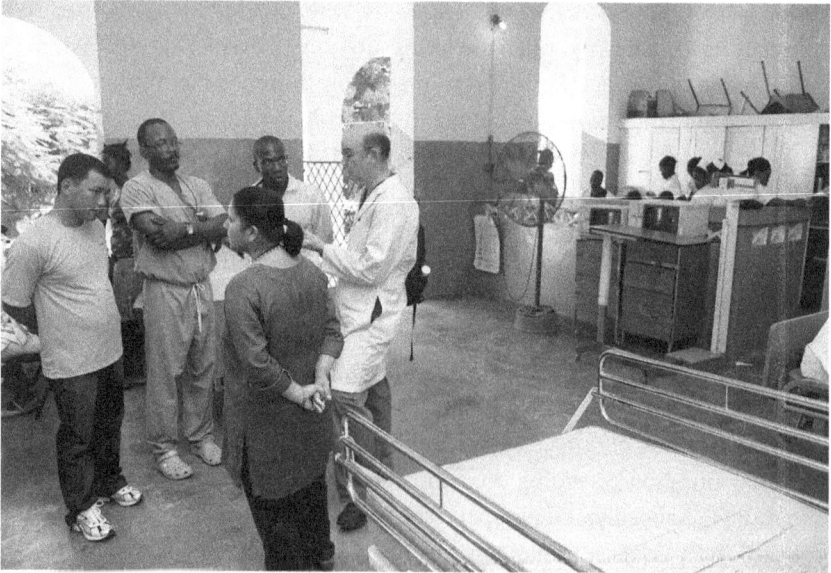

FIGURE 1.1.   An American doctor leads a tour of the Hôpital Universitaire Justinien's internal medicine department for two Nepalese UN physicians as part of an initiative to direct UN medical resources to the hospital. They are accompanied by two of the hospital's medical residents, both of whom speak excellent English. The hospital's administration chose not to participate in the tour. The nurses and nursing students (far right) were often excluded from international networking and partnerships. February 2009. Photo by Nathan Broaddus.

These issues are relatively visible to participants in the aid process, even if they often minimize their importance. I will now turn to some of the less obvious elements that have an influence on if and how medical aid is coordinated in the Haitian context. They are often invisible to casual observers and even to many of my informants, as they involve the subtle management of resources and priorities by actors involved in the aid process, and are often intentionally kept from public view.

"We Don't Have Anyone Else"

Several years ago, I was with a Haitian American director of a small medical aid NGO when she received a note from a local peasant woman, one she had helped with small gifts of money in previous years. The note, presumably written by someone else on the woman's behalf, described her many economic difficulties and pleaded for money for her children. The final line of the note read: "They'll tell you that we have other people who help us, but it's not true. We don't have anyone else, it's only you." Whether or not the woman did have another source of support (another foreigner, a relative in the diaspora, or a local benefactor) is not as remarkable as the fact that she felt compelled to explicitly disavow the possibility that she might. In considering why a visibly impoverished and desperate woman would make this claim when soliciting from a potential donor, one sees similar tendencies among the individuals, groups, and establishments that solicit and receive international medical aid, tendencies that have a direct impact on the coordination of this aid on a broader scale.

There are pressures to keep wealth and resources out of sight in Haiti, and these pressures apply to individuals of various social classes, as well as to organizations and establishments. Money is hidden behind high cement walls, stashed away in boxes or handkerchiefs, or spent through expenditures abroad.[5] One factor fueling this tendency is a fear of violent or forcible removal. While ordinary theft has long been an issue of concern in Haiti (*vòlè*, or thief, is among the worst insults used in Haiti, and it is used in a variety of contexts), the country experienced a dramatic increase in kidnappings for ransom beginning in the spring of 2005 (UNHCR 2008). The level of this type of crime has fluctuated over the past decade, and has led to significant fear and anxiety among middle- and upper-class Haitians in urban areas, particularly in and around Port-au-Prince.[6] Items such as expensive vehicles, elegant clothing and jewelry, and lavish home furnishings represent not only goods that could be taken but can also act as signals to potential thieves that the owner's family could mobilize a significant ransom if needed. I heard several Haitian health professionals talk about keeping their dress simple, driving an unremarkable vehicle, and avoiding being seen in expensive restaurants or hotels. One doctor chided me for using her professional title when addressing her as we traveled in a public bus together. Several of the hospital's residents had been kidnapped, assaulted, or shot during waves of instability that have intensified since 2005, and even if they had not been directly targeted, one of them told me, "all of us have been affected by the kidnappings in some way. All of us have family members or close friends who have been victims."

Public evidence or displays of wealth can also attract other forms of undesirable attention. While suspicions of jealousy and its place in illness etiology has received significant attention by medical anthropologists working in Haiti (Farmer 1992; Brodwin 1996), fewer have addressed the more visible and widespread practice of solicitation, in which individuals perceived to have resources or access to them are approached for support or assistance. Middle- and upper-class Haitians shield themselves from encounters with their more impoverished compatriots by restricting their movements to particular areas and spaces (specifically, private homes, workplaces, exclusive social spaces, and churches), by employing guards and security forces to restrict access to these spaces, and by riding in private vehicles whenever possible. In instances where they were directly solicited for funds in a public space (when entering or exiting churches and bakeries, for example), I observed physicians at times discretely slip a coin to the solicitor, or announce that they had no money with them.

In addition to keeping wealth hidden from those who would take or covet it, potential recipients also have reason to conceal existing wealth and resources from potential donors. This is particularly true in the case of international aid, and has a direct impact on its coordination or lack thereof. Aid groups and agencies working in Haiti often make explicit their intention to intervene among the poorest, neediest, and most neglected individuals and populations; in many cases, this intention is what spurred their initial interventions in Haiti. Haitians who are accustomed to working with these organizations and are familiar with their mandates take for granted that interventions directed at the most vulnerable and destitute will be of greatest appeal. When visiting establishments or communities with aid groups, I often saw and heard those soliciting aid, either for themselves, or on others' behalf, illustrate need in its various manifestations: a school without a roof, the reddish hair of a malnourished child, the absence of food in a kitchen. These needs were often described as greater or more extreme than any other in the area. While visiting a hospital with a group of potential donors from Canada, I overheard a physician tell the nurse guiding the group on their visit, "Don't be afraid to show them your bellybutton," in other words, the hospital's vulnerabilities and weaknesses. In this case, "bellybuttons" might include empty medicine cabinets, overcrowded hospital wards, and a lack of basic infrastructure. All of these could act as proof that aid was truly needed, and that the hospital was a worthy recipient. Because potential donors may turn away from potential recipients who already have resources (particularly those coming from external donors), those soliciting aid have an interest in concealing resources, or at least, keeping them discrete. A nurse told me that she believed that hospital administrators were letting one particular ward fall into a terrible state of decline with the hopes that an organization would be appalled by its condition, tear it down, and rebuild it.

These dynamics were particularly visible at the Justinien's Ophthalmology Department, which was renovated shortly before I began my research. Directed by a charismatic young physician who had completed her residency at the hospital and pursued further training in France, the department had received 160,000 USD from four international organizations to renovate its small building and purchase equipment and supplies. Visitors to the hospital often exclaimed, "Ophthalmology doesn't look like the rest of the hospital!" Not only was it clean, brightly painted, furnished with new equipment, and decorated with Haitian art but the department also had its own generator and small operating room, which granted it significant autonomy vis-à-vis the hospital's central administration. The department attracted patients from throughout northern Haiti, and was able to provide surgeries for cataracts, glaucoma, and other pathologies. The director, although visibly proud of her department's success, lamented that since its renovation, foreign visitors would take a quick look at Ophthalmology, compliment the service, and proclaim that it did not need their help before moving on to another section of the hospital. This was confirmed by several foreign volunteers and aid workers who told me that ophthalmology was not a priority for their organizations because of how well it was doing. Meanwhile, the department's staff hoped to attract new donors and to increase support from existing benefactors, as the number of patients seeking services had increased dramatically since the renovations. The department had also undertaken an ambitious project of eye screenings and mobile clinics in rural areas around Cap-Haïtien. The staff worried that their success might lead to their downfall, as new sources of support would probably continue to bypass them as long as their success was apparent. After hearing many narratives about the origins of diverse medical aid projects, which often involved an encounter with a crumbling clinic, an area void of medical services, or high rates of pathologies, it became clear to me that the solicitors and administrators of aid have good reason to avoid displaying their resources and strengths.

Paradoxically, pressures to hide existing wealth and resources are countered by incentives to do just the opposite: to display one's credentials as a dependable recipient of outside support, as one who has been entrusted in the past, and who is able to correctly manage future resources.[7] As much as donors seek out impoverished, needy, and neglected recipients, they are also eager to find deserving beneficiaries who are credible, competent, and, particularly in cases where aid is to be redistributed, able to allocate resources fairly and transparently. Haitian health professionals, who are often soliciting international aid on behalf of patients, are therefore obliged to present both pressing needs and evidence of success in helping address those needs. A particularly compelling strategy for achieving this balance is to recount or display instances in which previous support was discontinued or redirected, despite successes during the time of support. I often saw Haitian health professionals show foreign visitors buildings that fell into neglect, equipment that broke down, and empty pharmacies, all framed as evidence of prior support that was discontinued or had moved elsewhere. Not only do such displays highlight a current lack of support alongside evidence of preexisting capacities to absorb and redistribute aid but they can also be used to critique abandonment by prior supporters. It is all too easy to find evidence of discontinued, failed, and abandoned interventions in health establishments and other domains throughout Haiti, which is often described as a "graveyard of projects." Finally, visible affiliations with benefactors are also a source of prestige and status for Haitian recipients, who can use these relationships to earn admiration and respect.

Just as potential recipients have incentives to both hide and display the existence, provenance, and amount of resources they receive, donors are also caught between contradictory pressures to make their interventions visible and obvious and to conceal them and distribute in secrecy. The rewards of executing a very visible aid intervention are numerous. If the implementer of the intervention (whether foreign or Haitian) has received funds from another source, a public intervention will help protect the implementer from accusations of corruption or diverting funds. Elizabeth McAlister has described how aid in Haiti often operates in "the unseen world of hidden, covert, and sometimes illegal political and economic deals between both Haitians and Americans (and others) that have been instrumental in shaping the overlapping crises that Haitians confront" (McAlister 2010). Resources that are visibly distributed are more easily accounted for, and given the amount of aid funding and resources whose trajectories are not seen by the general public in Haiti or donor countries, a visible distribution is often a notable and remarkable event. Visible distributions of resources often occur in the context of public ceremonies, and are generally accompanied by speeches of gratitude and optimism. Even when distributions are not completely public, photographs are often used to increase the visibility of disbursement. The classic aid photograph shows donors and receivers smiling with the transferred resources—proof that they have indeed arrived.

A visible intervention may also prevent another actor from appropriating (or being credited by others for) the act. On several occasions during my fieldwork, individuals and foreign nongovernmental organizations were strongly encouraged by their Haitian partners to put their names and logos on material and infrastructure projects such as buildings, furnishings, and waste receptacles. In addition to deterring outright theft in the case of portable objects, donors were told that if their own identifying marker did not appear on the resource, people might think that the Haitian state had provided it. A stenciled name or logo would serve not only as a means for the donor to accumulate credit (Minn 2016) but also as a reminder to the population that the state was delinquent in its obligation to provide basic services. While foreign groups operating in Haiti are often accused of "planting their flags" for self-serving reasons (I concur that these accusations are often well-founded), I did observe cases in which it was the recipients, rather than the donors, who insisted that the latter's name appear on an intervention.

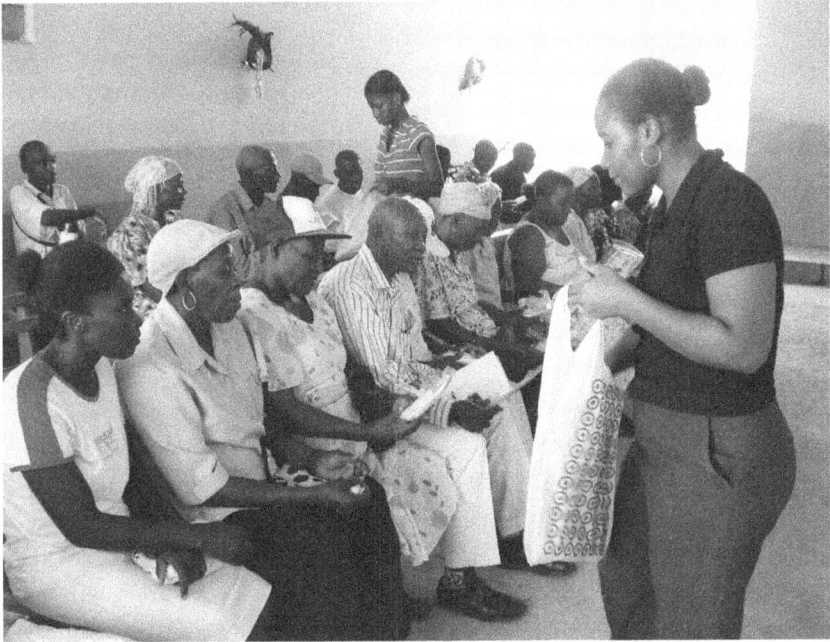

FIGURE 1.2.   The Haitian physician in the foreground of this image asked me to photograph her as she distributed the safe-birthing kits donated by a group of Americans. According to her, the photograph would assure the donors that their contributions were received by the intended beneficiaries. April 2009. Photo by the author.

There are pitfalls, however, when donors make their interventions visible, and some prefer to act in secrecy, complicating efforts at coordination. An important factor is the incapacity to respond positively to the numerous solicitations that a public distribution generally entails. The solicitations may be immediate, as in the case of a vitamin distribution or blood pressure screening that attracts large crowds. In these cases, there may be a great deal of excitement and fervor among the population hoping to access the resources, and while I have witnessed many such interventions take place harmoniously and without disruptions, being turned away because resources have run out can understandably lead to anger and agitation. Haitian health professionals and those foreigners with more experience in the country were often cautious about scheduling public distributions unless they were absolutely certain that their supplies would meet the demand. In some cases, security precautions were taken, including hiring men to act as security guards and restricting access to a distribution site by letting people through a barrier in small groups.[8]

In other cases, the solicitations that followed a visible intervention or distribution were not immediate, but were made at a later date. In the case of short-term visiting clinical teams, for example, the first two or three days of a weeklong mission tended to be quieter, but as word spread in the surrounding areas that foreign health workers were in the area, the number of patients grew, and on the final day, large crowds of hopeful patients had gathered near the site. (These trends were sometimes mitigated by local partners who began announcing the group's impending arrival in the preceding weeks, and in some cases distributed or sold cards that granted access to a consultation with the foreign team). On a smaller scale, individual group leaders described increases in individual solicitations after a visible intervention. Individuals or representatives from groups would appear at their hotels or guesthouses, often with a formal, written request for assistance. After the inauguration of the pediatrics emergency room was broadcast on Cap-Haïtien's radio station, the leader of an American NGO anticipated that the group would be heavily solicited because the organization's name was featured prominently at the inauguration ceremony and in subsequent radio reports. The same leader told me that he found turning down solicitations and requests to be one of the most difficult dimensions of his work in Haiti; this sentiment was echoed by many foreign aid workers and volunteers. They stressed that they consider the majority of requests to be reasonable (assistance for a school, medical supplies, food, housing, or basic infrastructure), and turning them down was therefore particularly discomfiting. As visible distributions tend to increase the number of subsequent solicitations, donors often preferred to keep their interventions discrete.

In short, understanding the coordination and lack of coordination of international medical aid in Haiti requires an awareness of the diverse and sometimes contradictory incentives participants in the aid process have to either make their actions and relationships publicly known, strategically visible to specific parties, or as concealed as possible. While most of my examples involve individuals and relatively small groups working in a very specific context, the pressures I have just described also exist on a larger scale, and can provide insights into the medical aid process in Haiti more broadly, as well as in other settings where the transfer of resources occurs in a context of great scarcity.

Dumping

In addition to the incentives that decrease the coordination of activities and interventions among the participants in international medical aid, there are other patterns and practices that have become naturalized as part of the aid process, and that are both the results and causes of a lack of coordination. I have grouped these practices under the umbrella term *dumping*, which is often used in formal economic terms to refer to predatory or heavily subsidized pricing. In the Haitian context, the term can be used to describe the influx of foreign commodities including food, used clothing and housewares, medications, and other items that have flooded even the most rural of markets in recent decades. Dumping has been identified as a contributing factor to food scarcity in Haiti, where local agriculture has been undermined by the arrival of cheap, heavily subsidized foreign foodstuffs. The most-cited example in this sphere is that of rice, which is imported to Haiti from the United States, undercutting Haitian farmers' prices and making the country's population vulnerable to fluctuations in price and food insecurity (Oxfam 2005). Other examples include white flour; frozen chicken backs, necks, and feet (parts of poultry generally not consumed in North America); secondhand clothing and shoes, which have reduced the demand for locally crafted apparel; motor vehicles and bicycles, which arrive to Haiti in varying states of disrepair; and housewares such as bedding, dishes, and furniture. Medicine and medical equipment also make their way to Haiti from other countries. In addition to the importation of pharmaceutical and medical products (primarily from India, Latin America, and China), medical goods also arrive in the form of donations from governments, NGOs, and pharmaceutical companies. These may be new, used, expired, or ambiguous in their condition and origin. As donations, they can be brought by the members of a group during their intervention, or dispatched by an overseas organization or agency to a Haitian or expatriate recipient.

There are two critiques inherent in the term *dumping*: one concerns the value or quality of the items in question, and the other is related to the means by which they are transferred. In the Haitian context, it is clear that many of the items which enter the country are of low or poor quality. White rice and flour offer little nutritional value, used clothes are often torn or stained (making them difficult to resell), and electronic equipment and machinery are often antiquated or barely functional. While these items are used throughout Haiti, and may have redeeming or appealing qualities (a market vendor once excitedly described to me how she had found four US dollars in the pocket of a donated shirt), they also represent Haiti's lack of local production and dependence on foreign nations for even the most basic of goods. In addition, even in the case of "free" donations or desirable items, their arrival and presence often create tense or potentially conflictual situations that recipients and administrators need to manage.

The second critique inherent in the term *dumping* lies in the way the item is transferred, that is to say, carelessly and indiscriminately. Dumping happens with little regard for when or where the item arrives, who benefits from (or is harmed by) it, or what the item's ultimate fate is. In the case of dumped aid, the items may arrive unannounced, or at a time when they are not needed, or when the labor or space needed to process or store the items is unavailable. The dumped items may have been sent to an inappropriate location, either in terms of local needs or inhospitable conditions. They may be targeted for a specific population that is not present at the site of delivery. Finally, dumped items are rarely followed-up on; the sender is not likely to make inquiries into their fate or address any of the issues or concerns that ensue from the dumping.

A case of dumping at the Justinien will illustrate some of these points. In the fall of 2008, a large shipping container of clothing, packaged food, medical supplies, and equipment arrived at the hospital. The container was sent by a foundation established by an American nurse, who named the foundation after herself, and appeared to be the only person involved in the organization. For the past five years, the nurse, who I will call Susan Miller, had been collecting donations to ship to countries in Africa, Asia, and Latin America. She had been moved to send the container to Haiti after seeing news reports of Haitians consuming mud "pies."[9] This container was the first she had sent to Haiti, and she traveled to Cap-Haïtien to be present for its arrival and unloading. When I met her in the hospital's courtyard, standing next to the container, she was extremely flustered and agitated. After asking about my presence and activities at the hospital, she asked if I would translate to facilitate her communication with the hospital administration. "Finally, someone who speaks English!" she exclaimed. She told me that she had been in touch with the hospital's administration by email, and that they were aware of her and the container's arrival, although this was refuted by the hospital staff I spoke with. Susan's main concern was to quickly get the container unloaded and distribute its contents. Her demeanor with the hospital staff was authoritative and impatient; she whispered to me that she suspected they were planning on stealing its contents: "There's a lot of corruption here!" she said. Meanwhile, the hospital administrators scrambled to find workers to unload the container, and find a space to store the donations. Their dismay with the situation was evident, and as I saw what was in the bags and boxes that began emerging, I could see why. The donations consisted of bags of wrinkled, used clothing, some of which appeared to be stained and torn; crumpled boxes of various medications and medical supplies, very little of it in intact packaging; and cases of sugary snacks and candies. There were several large bags of used stuffed animal toys, including an enormous purple Barney the Dinosaur plush figurine, which Susan claimed would be perfect for the pediatrics department. Finally, the shipment also included an antiquated colonoscope, which Susan warned was extremely fragile and valuable.

I spent much of the day with senior hospital administrators as they negotiated with Susan and attempted to find ways to deal with this large and unexpected donation. Their dilemma was representative of those experienced by many Haitians who act as nodes in international interventions. While Susan pushed for an immediate distribution of the clothes and food, the administrators feared that such an activity would attract a large number of hopeful recipients, and the hospital was already extremely crowded during ordinary periods of operation. Given the poor quality of the clothing, potential recipients might accuse them of having taken the best items for themselves. However, if they chose to discard the donations or direct them elsewhere, both the donor and the local population would be likely to accuse them of corruption, favoritism, waste, or irresponsibility. Their solution to the dilemma was to store the items in order to liberate and send away the shipping container, thereby placating Susan by demonstrating that the donations would be cared for, and ultimately postponing the decision about how to distribute the items. After deciding that much of the material could be stored in a covered stairwell (securing space, whether it be for clinical care, administrative work, or storage was one of the hospital's main challenges), two hospital porters began unloading the donations. As they became aware of what kinds of goods they had received, the hospital administrators became increasingly frustrated. Most of the clothing was deemed useless, the medical products appeared to them to be of dubious quality, and would demand a great deal of time and energy to sort through, and the colonoscope faced an uncertain future, as there were no personnel trained in colonoscopy techniques employed at the Justinien. (They also determined that Barney, with his imposing stature and gaping jaws, was likely to provoke more terror than comfort among the hospital's pediatric patients.) All of these assessments and the emotions they provoked were hidden from Susan, who dashed back and forth between the container and the storage room to make sure the process was going smoothly. The hospital staff also maintained hope that more useful items would appear from the depths of the shipping container, but when I spoke to them the following day, their assessment was that this particular donation had caused much more trouble than it was worth.

The critiques of dumping are quite different from another common critique of aid: that the materials or resources sent are insufficient. Informants frequently echoed the following statement from a hospital employee: "The little they do give you gets used up very quickly. It's as if they never give you enough to get you standing on your own two feet." Rather, in dumping, the primary critiques are not about the aid's insufficiency, but involve the poor quality of the items, the donor's lack of regard or consideration for the recipient of the aid, the ensuing life of the gift, and the consequences it may have on others. As one resident told me: "The people who give are satisfied to just give, but they don't really have oversight over what they've given." The case of expired medications is illustrative. In the last few decades, Haiti's Ministry of Health has become stricter about its policy that expired medications should not be allowed into the country. Working with customs officials and law enforcement agencies, this initiative has led to a greater number of incoming pharmaceuticals being confiscated and destroyed. Similarly, the Justinien's administration has implemented a policy of discarding medications from its depot that have reached their expiration dates, but must be careful about doing so, given that public knowledge of medicine being incinerated could bring about outrage in the local population. In such situations, it might be much easier for Haitian administrators and health personnel if the expired (or nearly expired) medications had not been sent in the first place, although donations of medicine from abroad represent an important weapon in the fight against morbidity and mortality in Haiti.

While much of the critique related to aid, coordination, and dumping expressed by Haitian informants was directed at international organizations, agencies, and governments, many also expressed a critical perspective about their own and their colleagues' role in receiving and administering aid. For example, a Haitian physician told me, "The people who receive aid distribute it poorly, they use it poorly. . . . We have things that are rotting in the depot, and when you prescribe medicine for a patient, they don't have money to buy it. They [the hospital administrators] only give out the medicine when it's expired." Almost invariably, critiques of foreigners' thoughtless and nefarious dumping practices were tied to the Haitian state's inability or unwillingness to control or prevent such practices. While Haitians have grown accustomed to their state's weaknesses and failures, they continue to assert that the state should assume its roles and responsibilities. Primary among these was the coordination of international actors in the country.

Coordination and the Haitian State

Within the Haitian government, there are two ministries that have a mandate to coordinate international medical aid: the Ministry of Public Health and Population (MSPP) and the Ministry of Planning and External Cooperation (MPCE). Foreign NGOs operating in Haiti are legally required to receive official status from the MPCE and those working in the health sector must obtain approval from the MSPP to conduct their activities. I encountered groups who had been waiting for several years to hear back from the ministries after having submitted their applications and forms. Many groups begin or continue their operations during this limbo period, and others, having witnessed other organizations' failure to receive a response to their applications, never initiate the registration process in the first place.

Like other ministries, the MPCE's and the MSPP's extreme centralization in Port-au-Prince means that local branch offices and representatives have little

authority or resources. While the northern branch office of MSPP in Cap-Haïtien held meetings, seminars, and trainings for the employees of public health
establishments throughout the department, to my knowledge, it never brought
together the various international groups and agencies active in the region the
way foreign-led initiatives have. For many of the groups that operate in Cap-Haïtien and other parts of northern Haiti, Port-au-Prince is simply a transit point
between a foreign destination and their site of intervention in Haiti. In recent
years, many groups have avoided the capital altogether because of insecurity and
the expense of lodging and transportation there. This, combined with the limited
capacity of departmental ministry offices to make executive decisions or grant
authorizations, means that many foreign organizations can and do avoid inter-
acting with state structures as much as possible.

Considering the Haitian government's potential role in coordinating aid
raises a number of complex issues. While Haiti has been governed by democrati-
cally elected governments for most of the last twenty-eight years, its long legacy
of dictatorships, coup d'états, and instability bring into relief the risks of rely-
ing on a fragile or "predatory" state (Fatton 2002). These risks have increased
with the uncertainty that accompanies decreasing voter turnout in Haiti, the
reestablishment of the Haitian army in 2017 (the army had been disbanded by
President Jean-Bertrand Aristide in 1995), and the assassination of President
Jovenel Moïse in July of 2021. In addition, coordination can very easily lead to
centralization, as well as the concentration of resources and authority, which
is frequently named as one of Haiti's major social and political problems. The
perils of centralization have been dramatically illustrated by the impact the 2010
earthquake has had on the country as a whole in terms of governance, the economy, and political instability. Examples of centralized resources and procedures
abound. The administrators at the Justinien (and at any public establishment
throughout the country) cannot hire, promote, or fire any of their personnel
at any level without the written approval of the Minister of Health in Port-au-
Prince. International aid (particularly that which is independently and locally
managed and negotiated) offers a wide variety of resources and possibilities
that are unavailable through the state. In many instances, it is evident why coordination and centralization would often be less appealing than autonomy and
flexibility.

Responsibility for Coordination

In the summer of 2008, a volunteer American physician who travels frequently
to a village near Cap-Haïtien sent an email to a dozen foreign and Haitian health

professionals active in the area to invite them to a meeting of what would become the Cap Haitien Health Network.[10] This internet-based group now has several hundred members. The group includes both North American health professionals involved in health projects in northern Haiti and Haitian health professionals, including the director of the MSPP's northern office, higher-level staff of hospitals in the region, and the employees or partners of international NGOs. The leader of the network organizes meetings three or four times a year in Cap-Haïtien, which are attended by foreign members who happen to be in the area at the time and Haitian and expatriate members who live in or near the city. In addition to meetings in Haiti, the network organizer created an internet listserve for members to share and request information. The listserve became particularly active in the aftermath of the 2010 earthquake and cholera epidemic, but its activities have decreased significantly in recent years.

I attended several of the network's meetings, which were usually held in one of Cap-Haïtien's more expensive hotels. At a typical meeting, approximately half of those in attendance were Haitian administrators, clergy, and medical professionals, and half were visiting American volunteers, primarily nurses and doctors, as well as two American NGO directors living in Haiti. A representative from each organization was asked to describe their group and its mission. After a few introductions, it became clear that despite the presence of the Haitian participants, the foreigners were the target audience for all the communication that was taking place. The comment that best exemplified this dynamic was from an American NGO director, who said to the group, "Whenever you're here in Haiti, I hope that you'll let me know, and we'll take you around to different communities."

The attendance at the meetings, while intended to include anyone working to address health issues in the area, represented a very specific segment of this larger group—namely, mid-level, professional individuals involved in international aid. By meeting in exclusive social spaces, and by communicating through foreign NGO networks and internet technology, the meeting effectively excluded individuals who lacked the appropriate contacts or social status. At the early meetings, no representatives from any of the area's three major hospitals or the MSPP were present. When I asked the network leader about their absence, he did not recognize the ministry's name, and told me that, for the hospital representatives, "I sent them an email inviting them, so they can't claim that they didn't know about it."[11] Conversely, there were a number of foreign volunteers present at these initial meetings who were on their first trip to Haiti and had limited knowledge about the activities of their own host organizations, and even less about health conditions or medical resources in the area.

While internet-based groups and networks such as the Cap Haitien Health Network will undoubtedly facilitate communication and coordination among certain individuals and groups, the extent to which they will affect coordination of international aid and Haitian-foreign partnerships more broadly remains to be seen. While internet access in Haiti has increased significantly in recent years, a substantial portion of the population remains functionally illiterate and unable to access computers or internet technologies. This may lead to new divides between those who have access to information, networks, and contacts and those who do not. In addition, access does not equal use, and I have heard both Haitians and foreigners complain that their email messages to overseas partners frequently go unanswered. With the multiplication of internet-based platforms, programs, and media for telecommunications and their enormous impact on individuals, relationships, and institutions, more empirical work is needed on how these technologies shape transnational processes and experiences in Haiti and other sites that have struggled for years with deficiencies in communications infrastructure.

Like Ramah McKay (2018), who found that the presence and influence of NGOs in Mozambique did not eclipse the state, the Haitian government remains an important provider of health services throughout the country. However, unlike the Mozambican government, its role as a "coordinator of interventions" (25) is minimal. McKay also notes that there is "widespread agreement in Maputo on the value of the public system"; no such agreement exists in Haiti. Many people stress the dysfunction or rot in the public system that would justify a revolution or a refounding of the Haitian state or other drastic measures. One American aid worker told me about being approached by a Haitian civic organization asking them to deliver their appeal to the US president to make Haiti the fifty-first American state. However, a widespread and persistent outcry about the state's failure to serve its citizens by Haitians of all social classes suggests the endurance of claims made on this same state. This dynamic appears to be similar to that found by Adia Benton (2015) in her examination of HIV/AIDS prevention and care programs in Sierra Leone: "To emphasize a state's inability to provide social welfare and care for its members presumes a natural function of the state. Even as a state 'fails' in its perceived responsibilities, it remains a potent fantasy in its members' claims for justice and aspirations to live moral lives" (136).

The relationships between nongovernmental actors, foreign governments and the Haitian state can be considered in terms of sovereignty. In 2002 Mariella Pandolfi coined the term *mobile sovereignties* to characterize NGOs and international organizations that, through their actions and operations, "impose institutions and concepts of citizenship that are alien to territories in which the nation-state has never established its power" (Pandolfi 2002, 34). In order to do so, these groups use a wide range of means, but rely on existing power structures. The moving sovereignties constitute "a network of governance characterized by innovative strategies of de- or re-territorialization" (35). For Pandolfi, the "humanitarian apparatus," acts on three levels: the right to intervene, the temporality of emergency, and the imperative to act. Humanitarian work, she argues, is fundamentally homogenizing, creating interchangeable categories such as "the trafficked woman" or "the refugee child."

Pandolfi's framework cannot be applied to Haiti in blanket terms. Growing partnerships between NGOs and the Haitian state, for example, complicate the distinction between these two categories. However, many of her categories—developed during fieldwork in the aftermath of the Balkan conflicts—do apply to the Caribbean nation, confirming again that Haiti is not an exceptional case, but rather indicative of larger global patterns. The language of emergency or crisis is certainly invoked in Haiti, both within the country and by outside observers (Beckett 2019). The Haitian state's incapacity to coordinate foreign aid and the interventions on its national territory certainly demonstrates the limits of its sovereignty, limits that are tied to the geopolitical and economic interests of powerful state and nonstate actors. In addition to the presence of hundreds of NGOs working in various sectors throughout the country, Haiti has also been the site of a number of UN missions since 1993, notably MINUSTAH, the UN Mission for the Stabilization of Haiti. Established after Jean-Bertrand Aristide's ouster in 2004, the multinational force was composed of soldiers and officers from various countries, with strong representations of Latin American, Asian, and Middle Eastern contingents. The mission officially ended in 2017, but was immediately replaced by MINUJUSTH, a nonmilitarized peacekeeping mission, and BINUH, the United Nations Integrated Office in Haiti, which had its mandate renewed until July of 2022.

The enormous influx of international aid that entered Haiti in the aftermath of the January 2010 earthquake, compounded with the damage to Haitian state infrastructures and the uncertainty related to the upcoming change in government portend that coordination will continue to be a major issue. If the various parties who have called for increased coordination are sincere in their stated desires, they will have to take into consideration their own and others' motivations and incentives for not coordinating, and make serious attempts to mitigate their negative effects. One of the most challenging dimensions of coordinating medical aid is that it involves so many different components: institutions, individuals, material goods, intangible services, and financial resources. In the following chapter, I will examine the work of a specific medical aid organization to illustrate the challenges even the most reflexive organizations face in trying to achieve their goals.

"WORKING TOGETHER FOR HEALTH" AT THE HÔPITAL UNIVERSITAIRE JUSTINIEN

The laundry service at the Hôpital Universitaire Justinien is located behind the hospital's oldest and largest building, the internal medicine wing. In contrast to the building's thick, whitewashed walls, graceful arches, and terra-cotta roof tiles, the laundry service is reminiscent of the shacks and lean-tos in Cap-Haïtien's shantytowns, with its corrugated metal roof and flimsy wooden pillars. The lack of walls does allow breezes from the adjacent hillside to push aside the stifling, humid heat, however, and there are fewer mosquitoes here than in the hospital's closed buildings. On a typical afternoon, six women ranging in age from sixteen to late sixties are seated on low chairs in front of two worn cement basins the size of large bathtubs. They pound sticks of harsh, beige soap into balls the size of oranges and painstakingly lather their way through the piles of sheets, surgical drapes, and hospital scrubs that are brought to the laundry in wheelbarrows every morning. An elderly male employee is responsible for filling the basins from nearby spigots or, more often, with water hauled in large buckets from a well on the other side of the hospital grounds. I would often stop and visit the laundresses during the downtimes in my research, between meetings with foreign medical teams or after interviews with medical residents. All of the laundry's employees had moved to the city of Cap-Haïtien from surrounding villages, and we often talked about the economic hardships that had forced them to move to the city and their nostalgia for life in a quieter, gentler environment. Having spent my first months in Haiti in such a village, I was happy to find familiar modes of joking and storytelling that contrasted with more formal interactions with physicians and nurses. The laundresses told me that they were happy to have a visitor since they felt mostly ignored by the hospital's leadership and its steady stream of dignitaries and foreign visitors, who seemed to pay attention to the hospital's lower-level employees only if there were manual tasks that needed to be done or if these employees went on strike.

While family members are expected to wash patients' clothes and bring bedding and towels from home, the laundry service is responsible for washing surgical drapes from the operating room, the scrubs of lower-level employees (physicians and nurses are responsible for maintaining their own gowns and scrubs), and bedding from the postsurgery recovery room. As I sat talking with the laundresses, the washing water would turn crimson from clots of blood in the clothes and sheets. Unfazed, they continued to scrub at the fabric, squeezing it so tightly that jets of water sprayed out between their fingers. While most of the items they washed were made of cotton, they also cleaned sheets and drapes made of thin plastic. These are intended for single use but, in a context of ongoing and extreme scarcity, will be reused many times until they tear and shred. Ironically, the nonabsorbent plastic is much easier to wash than cloth, as it has no fibers to absorb blood or other fluids.

The laundry service at the Justinien represents different things to different individuals. For the laundresses themselves, the work is repetitive, tiring, and poorly paid, but regular, long-term employment is extremely difficult to find in Haiti, and these women have few alternatives that would entice them to leave their work. For the hospital's directors and professional employees, the laundry is an essential but undesirable service. They know that hospitals in what they often refer to as *les pays organisés* (the organized countries) rely on electric and automated washing, drying, and sterilization for linens or dispose of single-use items according to the manufacturer's instructions. For the members of Konbit Sante, one of the many international aid organizations that provide aid to the Justinien, the laundry has been both an object of intervention and a site for learning a cautionary tale about the unexpected consequences of aid. In this chapter, I analyze the work of Konbit Sante, a small, secular American organization and draw on the group's struggles to "build capacity" in Haiti's public health system. In choosing not to provide clinical services to Haitian patients, Konbit Sante joins a growing number of organizations and agencies that have been shaped by long-standing critiques of humanitarian and development practices. In describing the Konbit Sante's struggles to maintain partnerships with their Haitian colleagues, I illustrate the persistence of gift relations in global health, and the tensions that arise as actors negotiate between material and immaterial forms of aid. I argue that, despite donors' and recipients' desire to distances themselves from donations of material supplies, these types of donations often create the necessary conditions for systemic and structural interventions that are increasingly identified as global health priorities.

Konbit Sante: Working Together for Health

Konbit Sante was founded in 2000 by a group of health professionals in Portland, Maine.[1] While several nurses, public health specialists, and physicians were involved in creating the group, the dermatologist Michael Taylor and his wife, Wendy Taylor, a marketing researcher, are considered to be the organization's founders and its driving force in its early years. Unlike organizations founded by Haitians who had migrated overseas or by individuals living in areas with a significant Haitian population, Konbit Sante's decision to work in Haiti came not from a prior connection with the country, but from a more generalized desire to "do something" in a place that needed it. The group chose to work in Haiti after considering sites in Africa and Central America, which were deemed too distant for regular interventions. A chance contact with a physician from northern Haiti led to a visit by a delegation from Portland to Cap-Haïtien in 2001 and the identification of the Justinien as a potential site of intervention. The arbitrariness of this choice and the identification of a potential recipient population based on perceived need rather than national affinities or other preexisting ties are not uncommon in global health. Many of the relationships that form among individuals and organizations in global health initiatives develop among strangers through chance encounters or coincidences—meeting an individual from the area in question, or seeing a news report about a population in need, for example. The apparent arbitrariness of these origin stories in global health or humanitarian projects stands in contrast with those that emerge out of kin or diasporic support networks, and can sometimes lead to questions about donors' motivations and sincerity.

Another striking feature of Konbit Sante was the fact that many of its founding members had already been involved in overseas medical aid initiatives and formed the organization in response to dissatisfaction with existing models of aid. Several among them, including the Taylors, had participated in short-term international medical missions, a common type of intervention whereby clinicians from wealthy countries travel to poorer ones with pharmaceutical products and biomedical equipment to treat underserved populations. Medical missions may collaborate with preexisting hospitals or health centers, but often set up temporary clinics in schools or churches. While these missions can reach patients who would otherwise be unable to access biomedical services and treatments, they have been criticized for undermining existing health systems, providing only short-term care, and catering more to the desires of volunteers than to the health needs of impoverished populations (Maki et al. 2008; Sykes 2014; Unite for Sight 2016).

The founders of Konbit Sante, well aware of these weaknesses, told me that they became frustrated by seeing the same populations with the same health problems year after year during their annual trips. Out of this frustration emerged a new model of intervention, one based on the decision not to facilitate clinical care for Haitian patients by North American clinicians. Unlike the staff and volunteers of nearly all North American medical NGOs operating in Haiti, the members of Konbit Sante do not provide consultations, treatments, or surgeries for patients, even though most of the group's US-based staff and volunteers have been clinicians. Instead, the group's stated mission is to "support the development of a sustainable health system to meet the needs of the Cap-Haïtien community with maximum local direction and support." Its main activities include facilitating infrastructure projects, providing administrative and logistical support to the Haitian hospitals' and clinics' leadership teams, supporting education and training for Haitian clinicians, and facilitating donations of material supplies from North American donors.

Another of the group's distinguishing features is its relationship to the Haitian public health system. Since its inception in 2000, Konbit Sante has always worked explicitly in partnership with Haiti's Ministry of Health and Population (MSPP) and public health establishments, rather than with private hospitals or institutions. While the group cooperates with other NGOs and some private health care facilities, all of its activities and interventions take place with and through the public sector. This is in contrast to many other NGOs, whose partnerships with the Haitian government appear to be reluctant compromises borne of necessity, convenience, or donor pressures. Many foreign NGOs, particularly smaller organizations, operate autonomously from the Haitian government and are intentional in their efforts to avoid the latter. Konbit Sante is explicit in its mission to avoid creating a "parallel health care system," even though its members and volunteers openly state that partnering with the Haitian government is burdensome and significantly slows the pace at which interventions are implemented. This commitment to strengthening Haiti's public health system emerges from the group's founders' vision of public health and the role of the state in providing health services. Many Konbit Sante members, including its former executive director, Nathan (Nate) Nickerson, have worked within the public health sector in Maine and elsewhere in the United States.

Finally, Konbit Sante is unusual in that it intervenes only in northern Haiti, specifically in Cap-Haïtien and its surrounding area. The majority of the group's activities take place at the Justinien, but it is also active at the Hôpital de Fort-St-Michel, a smaller hospital located in the outskirts of Cap-Haïtien. Most foreign organizations of Konbit Sante's size operate either in rural areas or in Port-au-Prince, while larger organizations often work at multiple sites throughout the country.

Although most of its activities are hospital-based, Konbit Sante's interventions over the past twenty years have been extremely diverse. They have taken place in nearly all of the Justinien's twelve departments, as opposed to other organizations that form partnerships with single departments and, often, with a specific single clinician in that department.[2] Konbit Sante's activities include providing salary supplements for physicians to improve the quality of resident supervision, implementing infrastructure projects to improve the hospital's electricity and water systems, obtaining funds to renovate and expand hospital buildings, shipping large containers of donated medical supplies from Maine and setting up an electronic database to track the use of the materials, and facilitating collaborative research between Haitian and American clinicians. When I interviewed Haitian medical staff at the HUJ to talk about their experiences with international aid, they nearly always began by describing the work of Konbit Sante. The hospital's directors often referred to the organization as their *partenaire privilégié* (our privileged or favored partner) to distinguish them from the many other groups and agencies that provided aid to the hospital.

While Konbit Sante is in many ways an exceptional organization, it can also be considered in terms of larger trends in the global health movement that has emerged over the past three decades. As a form of biomedical humanitarianism, Konbit Sante embodies many of the characteristics and values that are prominent in global health, including the promotion of rights-based discourses about health, a focus on health disparities, and the prominence of partnerships between state and nonstate actors to provide health services. In addition, Konbit Sante is a US-based and US-led organization; like so many of the institutions, foundations, and universities that drive global health initiatives, its identity emerges out of both an American Judeo-Christian heritage of faith-based charity and a more secular tradition of civic-minded voluntary action. In this sense, Konbit Sante resembles a much larger and more prominent New England-based organization working in Haiti, Partners in Health (PIH). PIH's model and the work of its founder, the physician-anthropologist Paul Farmer, were influential in Konbit Sante's formative years, as several of Konbit Sante's leaders were impressed and inspired by PIH's work and met with Farmer and other PIH staff to discuss the direction Konbit Sante would take. The organizations operate in distinct geographic areas and on different scales: PIH employs more than six thousand people—primarily Haitian nationals—for its Haiti projects and, in

2015, spent nearly a third of its 133.7 million USD budget in that country alone. Konbit Sante has a dozen employees and an annual budget of just over 1.5 million USD. However, both organizations focus on reducing health inequalities, building capacity among Haitian medical staff, and working with the Haitian government.

My efforts to understand Konbit Sante's work and the relationships it develops with Haitian clinicians were greatly facilitated by its members' self-reflexivity. More than most other groups I studied, its members frequently questioned the efficacy, impact, and consequences of their interventions and did so openly with both Haitian and non-Haitian interlocutors. Their interventions tend to be designed with great caution and deliberation, lacking the inflection point of emergency and crisis that is so present in humanitarian logic (Pandolfi 2002; Calhoun 2008). One of my earliest encounters with Nate Nickerson involved a cautionary tale about the laundry service I just described. During my first interview with Nate in 2006, he told me how Konbit Sante volunteers had obtained the donation of an industrial washing machine in 2004, after having witnessed the laborious (and potentially biohazardous) process of hand-washing linens in the hospital's laundry. The large machine was sent to the Justinien in a shipping container at great expense, but was used for only several days before the hospital administration reverted to the original system, leaving the washing machine in a state of disuse for the next decade.[3] It was eventually put to use in 2013 to wash only the most soiled of linens, while the laundresses continued to hand-wash the majority of sheets, drapes, and scrubs. Nickerson told me, "Whenever people in Maine talk about making a new donation or a new project, we always tell them about the washing machine and the lessons we learned during that whole process." The washing machine began as a failed gift, one that both donors and recipients had initially agreed would be valued and useful, but that would not be truly received and implemented in its full capacity for many years.

The washing machine, with its initial failure and eventual operation, is emblematic of both the material and intangible dimensions of international medical aid. As a nonmedical device whose main purpose is to ensure the hygiene of peripheral medical material (linens and surgical garments), the washing machine highlights the materiality of biomedical environments, references the labor (both mechanized and human) required to maintain hygienic clinical spaces, and indexes the inequalities—often gendered—between those who clean clothes by pressing buttons and those who must manually scrub soiled fabric for hours on end. For the leaders of Konbit Sante, donations like the washing machine represent a sort of compromise between the systemic changes in function and management they hope to engender at the hospital and the material donations they continue to send to Haiti in recognition of the tangible scarcities at the hospital and the impact these scarcities have on employees' morale and patients' health. The group has not compromised, however, on its early decision to forgo interventions on another category of material objects: patients' bodies.

Eschewing the Clinical

As I mentioned earlier, a defining feature of Konbit Sante is its lack of emphasis on the provision of clinical services by foreign staff and volunteers. This is in striking contrast to many of the small North American medical aid organizations that send teams to Haiti, some of which focus nearly exclusively on carrying out clinical interventions. The foreign medical workers involved with these teams (including nurses, physicians, pharmacists, physical therapists, and others) typically come to Haiti for a week to ten days every year to carry out consultations and various medical procedures. In rural areas with limited medical infrastructure, their activities may include routine checkups, distribution of medications (such as analgesics, antihypertensive drugs, and antiparasitic medications), screenings and referrals for pregnant women, wound care, and basic laboratory analyses. In situations where foreign organizations are partnered with larger Haitian health care establishments and more resources are available, teams may come to Haiti to perform specialized procedures on patients who have been pre-identified and preselected for operations.[4] Oftentimes, these organizations focus on a specific medical condition, such as cleft palate, club foot, or cataracts. Konbit Sante is explicit in its choice not to carry out clinical interventions. In the "How You Can Help" section of its website, its "Volunteers" page opens with the statement:

> Our model is different from many other groups in that we do not have regular volunteer positions/placements and our volunteers are not generally engaged in providing direct service while in Haiti. Instead, volunteers work in committees with staff and their Haitian colleagues to study needs, develop and implement initiatives, conduct trainings, make infrastructure improvements, and deliver much-needed equipment and supplies. (Konbit Sante n.d.)

The group's members are similarly explicit in describing Konbit Sante's decision not to provide clinical services. As one volunteer told me: "In contrast to many other groups that go to Haiti and that have an approach of going to take care of patients, that's not what we're about. We are trying to help build: build a health system." During the years I have spent at the HUJ, I was aware of only one instance in which a Konbit Sante member provided clinical services that were not oriented toward training Haitian staff. This situation involved a Portland-based surgeon who enjoyed operating with a Haitian surgeon at the HUJ as a way of cementing a bond of friendship between the two. His activities were considered peripheral to the organization's mission by Konbit Sante's leaders, who explained to me that they routinely turn down requests from North American clinicians seeking opportunities to travel to Haiti to offer medical services.

While the decision not to provide clinical interventions is a key part of Konbit Sante's identity as an organization, it is also the cause of confusion to outsiders. Nate Nickerson told me that he spends a lot of time explaining this model to people both in the United States and Haiti, who "don't always know how to categorize us." It is clear that most small NGOs that send volunteers to Haiti tend to focus on service provision. Konbit Sante, in its efforts to "work with existing structures to strengthen available health resources," not only challenges widespread assumptions by both Haitians and North Americans that foreign medical professionals in Haiti are there to provide clinical services but also engages in activities which are difficult or impossible to measure using funders' metrics and scales. Nickerson often told me that "funders want to know how many 'widgets' you've given out—we just don't work that way, and they don't know what to do with us." "Widgets" might refer to vaccines, eyeglasses, HIV therapies, crutches, or any of the many other countable items that are dispensed by most aid groups in Haiti. Although Konbit Sante does provide the hospital with a significant quantity of tangible material goods and while many of its nonclinical activities do have some quantifiable dimensions (for example, paying the salary of a physician who oversees the training of a specific number of medical residents), much of its work is difficult to convey in a field where clinical services have historically been and continue to be the currency through which interventions are measured and evaluated (Minn 2016). Conversely, this approach has also won the group supporters, particularly individuals who for various reasons are critical of existing models of international medical aid in Haiti and wish to invest in alternative strategies.

Konbit Sante's decision to forgo the provision of clinical services was also interpreted in different ways by the hospital's personnel. I was told several times by the HUJ's Haitian staff that the hospital did not host visiting teams of specialists because there was no designated lodging for them.[5] Many foreigners volunteering or working at the Justinien (including Konbit Sante's North American staff and volunteers) lodged at nearby hotels in Cap-Haïtien, which resulted in a significant expense for repeat travelers. Eventually, the organization rented an apartment for its visiting staff and volunteers. The Justinien's inability to house foreign medical teams is an example of the ways in which Haitian institutions—particularly government institutions—are said to lack the capacity to absorb outside resources. Foreign groups traveling to volunteer in Haiti often prioritize secure lodging and access to safe food and water near their site of intervention. Private and religious institutions that receive groups of volunteers from overseas often operate small guesthouses or dormitories; however, this is not the case for public institutions.

In choosing not to provide clinical services, Konbit Sante turned away from what informants from other organizations described to me as the most satisfying, rewarding, and tangible benefits of their involvement in Haiti: participating in the direct care and healing of individual patients, many of whom had serious medical conditions and few options for effective treatment. In knowing that they had prescribed antibiotics to cure an infant's potentially life-threatening infection, helped recover the sight of a young market woman, or repaired a hernia that would allow a rural farmer to continue working his land, most foreign medical volunteers in Haiti had constant, tangible rewards for their efforts. These rewards provide satisfaction and a sense of accomplishment in a setting where progress in the health sector more broadly often seems impossible, slow, or nonexistent. Konbit Sante, on the other hand, functions in another register of intervention, aiming for changes at a more systemic level. However, even when removed from the care of individual patients, material interventions continue to occupy an important place in Konbit Sante's work. They can act as catalysts (or crutches, if one espouses a critical perspective) for less tangible structural and administrative changes in the hospital's functioning. The success or failure of the subsequent partnerships was directly related to the provision or absence of material gifts as part of the intervention.

"They Do Not Come as Conquerors"

The pediatrics service at the Justinien consists of six inpatient rooms divided by patient age (neonates to adolescents), an outpatient clinic, and a malnutrition clinic (the latter two each consist of a single, small room). The service has an official capacity to intern approximately sixty patients, although it is not uncommon to find more than one patient in a bed. It officially employs nine attending physicians, twenty-three nurses and auxiliaries, and fifteen support staff, although many of the attending physicians rarely come to the service (absenteeism is less common among nurses and other staff). Sixteen residents account for the bulk of physician presence in the service. Most pediatric patients are accompanied by at least one family member, who provides food and bedding and often sleeps on the cement floor next to the patient's bed. It is not unusual for there to be an abandoned patient in at least one of the rooms—poverty and desperation drive parents or relatives to slip out of the service during the night, leaving the young patient dependent on the compassion of the medical staff or the other families nearby.[6] Because of the difficulties and costs involved in coming to the HUJ, which often include traveling long distances, sacrificing income-generating activities, and paying for consultation and medications at the hospital, parents are often unable to bring their child to the hospital or delay seeking treatment until the sickness has reached an advanced stage. Pediatric patients at the HUJ suffer from the largely preventable pathologies that afflict children throughout Haiti: diarrheal diseases, respiratory infections, malnutrition, and infectious diseases.

Pediatrics is the service at the HUJ where Konbit Sante has been the most active. This can be evaluated by the scope and quantity of resources dispensed, the number of volunteers involved, and the frequency of meetings and interventions with members of the service. A key component of Konbit Sante's work in the pediatrics service involves medical residents. When the organization began its work at the hospital, a single resident was being trained in pediatrics. This was unanimously attributed to a lack of training and mentorship available from staff physicians, who demonstrate high rates of absenteeism. With no staff mentors, set curriculum, or specific training opportunities, pediatrics at the Justinien had limited appeal for medical students choosing residency programs. In 2005 Konbit Sante agreed that it would supplement the salary of a staff physician who would be responsible for and take an active role in training residents. By the time I completed my research at the hospital, the number of residents had grown to sixteen, and a second physician had been hired by Konbit Sante and the hospital to help train the residents. Other pediatric health workers employed by the organization include a nurse educator at the hospital's affiliated nursing school and two community health agents who provide follow-up care and visits to infants discharged from the Justinien's pediatric inpatient malnutrition program.

Konbit Sante's interventions in pediatrics also include tangible forms of material assistance. The organization funded the remodeling and renovation of the pediatrics conference room, where morning reports, residents' academic presentations, and other meetings take place. Konbit Sante procured and delivered all the furniture in the room (used but functional tables, chairs, and shelving from hospitals in Maine) as well as a variety of textbooks, a television monitor, a projector, and computers. In the pediatric intensive care units, Konbit Sante installed the tubing and spigots necessary to provide oxygen to multiple infants, replacing the previous system where infants received oxygen directly from a single tank.[7] In addition to renovating and developing existing spaces, Konbit Sante solicited funds from outside donors to build a pediatric outpatient consultation room and, most recently, a pediatric emergency room. The head pediatrician's speech at the room's inauguration hints at both the appreciation HUJ employees feel for Konbit Sante and the expectations they have for future support:

> They do not come as conquerors. They don't impose any orders, any pre-existing conditions, any constraints. The name they have chosen for their organization is telling. Konbit Sante favors the effective participation of all actors involved in a colossal collective work. Success on the ground and good results are their only motivations and often the only guarantees that they require from their partners. We must come together to achieve a single and essential goal: health in all its dimensions. As proof of this philosophy, this approach, this room will allow us in pediatrics to improve and modernize the quality of the care we give. An emergency room today, soon an intensive care unit, a neo-natology service, a dormitory for the patients' families.

This physician is well-known among Konbit Sante's US-based staff and volunteers for his manifold and repeated requests for aid for the pediatrics service. Some who were present for the speech chuckled at hearing the proposal for new projects that accompanied the appreciation for one that had just been completed.

Haitian and American participants in Konbit Sante's activities offered several theories to explain the group's marked presence and success in the pediatric service. Foremost among them was that donors are particularly moved by and likely to intervene in the health needs of children. This would explain the strong presence of Konbit Sante and other international groups in pediatrics as compared to departments such as urology and dentistry. Such tendencies reflect larger patterns. In her work on gifts in India, Erica Bornstein (2010) has described the significance of children, particularly orphaned children, in humanitarian discourse. Similarly, Liisa Malkki (2010, 59) claims that the figure of the child does "ritual and affective work [in] transnational representational spheres," including its embodiment of human goodness and the future and its role as a prototypical sufferer. Sick children are the ideal recipients of aid. They are defined by their needs and not expected to reciprocate because they are thought to have nothing to give back. Giving to children operates on another level. In her subsequent writing about "trauma teddies," and "aid bunnies," Malkki (2015) describe how handmade toys sent to children around the world in the context of humanitarian aid interventions provide a sense of connection to the world and to children in need for knitters in the global North who may be elderly and lonely.

Another factor has been the personalities and characteristics of the individuals involved in the partnership. As I just mentioned, the head of the pediatric service has been consistently eager for new collaborations and projects. His demeanor toward foreign partners is friendly and enthusiastic, and he regularly presents long lists of needed materials, renovations, and constructions to Konbit Sante and other potential donors. On the American side, several pediatricians and pediatric nurses have been particularly active in traveling to Haiti and procuring donated materials, supplies, and funding from American health establishments and donors. Despite Konbit Sante's efforts to work throughout the hospital's various departments, the inception and success of its activities often depend heavily on the interests and availability of its American members. In some cases, however, even interest and availability are not enough to secure a successful partnership. This was the case for the hospital's nursing department.

"They Should Stop Pushing So Hard"

Over the years, many of Konbit Sante's programs have developed when health professionals from Maine approach personnel from the corresponding medical specialty at the Justinien and initiate dialogue that they hope will lead to fruitful collaborations.[8] Nurses have been prominent and active in Konbit Sante since the organization's inception. Nate Nickerson, in addition to holding a doctorate in public health, is also a registered nurse, and asserts this occupational identity proudly. Nurses are also active on the organization's board and in its various committees and are nearly always present during group trips to Cap-Haïtien. In 2006 several nurses in the organization began considering the possibility of developing a formal partnership with the nurses at the hospital. From conversations with nurses and other hospital staff, they concluded that nurses at the Justinien shoulder heavy responsibilities, are underpaid and underappreciated, and face some of the similar inequalities in status and power vis-à-vis physicians as do their American counterparts. In addition to reporting to the director of their respective services, nurses at the Justinien work under the supervision of a head nurse in each service, who in turn reports to the director of the Bureau de Nursing, a nurse named Mis Louis.[9] In planning to establish a partnership with the nurses at the hospital, the North American nurse members of Konbit Sante approached Mis Louis and the other members of the hospital's administrative council. Reactions to the original proposal were positive, and meetings between the American and Haitian nurses were planned for dates when the former would be in Cap-Haïtien.

I sat in on several of these meetings, which usually included Mis Louis, the executive director of Konbit Sante, two or three visiting American nurse volunteers, and the head nurses from various departments throughout the hospital. Almost all of the hospital's departments were represented, and those who were late were called by their colleagues and encouraged to hurry. The meetings

I attended shared a similar format. The Haitian nurses were asked to describe what they envisioned a partnership with Konbit Sante might look like and what the organization could do to make their work easier. Their discourses were fairly consistent and focused on lack of medical materials, understaffing, and problems with material infrastructure such as electricity, water, and space. The American nurses acknowledged these challenges, but from prior conversations with them, I knew that they did not want to focus on providing materials or supplies and did not want to add major infrastructure projects to those already undertaken by the organization. During the meetings, the tension was palpable. The Haitian nurses sat with their arms crossed, looking at the floor or at the desk in front of them. The American nurses leaned forward, anxiously listening and looking for signs and communication. All the questions and statements were translated between Creole and English either by me or by Konbit Sante's regular translator, which added to the length of the meetings. The meetings ended on a note of uncertainty, with promises to follow up on specific procedural items but no conclusive agreements about projects or activities that would raise the enthusiasm of the participants.

After one of these awkward encounters, a Haitian nurse who had a positive rapport with members of Konbit Sante and believed that the American nurses were acting in good faith told me, "They should stop pushing so hard. The nurses here will think that they're getting money to work with us, and that's why they're so insistent on developing a partnership." Ironically, the American nurses' sense of professional solidarity with their Haitian counterparts and their strong commitment to establishing a partnership made the Haitian nurses suspicious of them. This was not the first or only time I encountered Haitian recipients (active or potential) who interpreted donors' zeal as evidence of an ulterior, self-interested motivation for providing aid. Donors were rarely aware of such interpretations, and if they did become aware of them, some concluded that Haitians "do not understand altruism."[10]

Over the course of many months and after several meetings in Haiti, discouraged by what they perceived as a lack of enthusiasm or initiative by the Haitian nurses and at a loss to know what a potential partnership could involve in concrete terms, the American nurses set aside the project for a nursing partnership between Konbit Sante and the Justinien. While both Haitian and American nurses continue to play important roles in the organization and its programs, a formal partnership centered on nurses was never formed.

The differences in outcomes between the pediatrics partnership and the anticipated nursing partnership have multiple causes. As opposed to pediatrics—which is a specific department that is structured by a single hierarchy and operates within a clearly defined physical space—nursing is diffused throughout the hospital and is not as united by physical or hierarchical structures. In addition, it is more difficult to garner international support and resources for nurses than for infants and children. A final factor is the role of material aid in the two partnerships. Because Konbit Sante's nurses had nothing tangible to offer, no materials that would make the Justinien's nurses' work easier or their shifts more comfortable, it was difficult for the former's initiatives for partnership to gain traction. The oxygen tubing, textbooks, and emergency room that acted as goodwill ambassadors in the pediatrics department and paved the way for more structural interventions in that department, had no equivalent for the nursing service.

Persistent Gifts

In their critique of material aid as an unsustainable "Band-Aid" solution that undermines lasting and systemic changes, Konbit Sante's members echo those of prominent critics of development and aid, who have called into question the large-scale transfer of economic resources and material from wealthy to impoverished areas. Economists' critiques about the failures of international aid have argued that conventional aid programs (including material donations) lead to dependency, market distortion, corruption, and ultimately worsening conditions for the aid's intended recipients (Easterly 2006; Moyo 2009). These critiques are intended to dispel the commonly held assumption that international aid helps the world's poorest population.

Critics of aid must confront the fact that material gifts often garner immediate enthusiasm and satisfaction among both donors and recipients. At the Justinien, many donations serve basic and immediate needs: pharmaceutical products treat ailments, bandages protect wounds, chairs provide a place for patients and staff to sit. Because of the centrality of material objects in biomedical diagnostics and treatment, the equipment and products sent by Konbit Sante contribute in unambiguous ways to the practice of biomedicine in Haiti. Donated items are omnipresent throughout the hospital, and the Haitian staff and patients regularly request additional material goods from visiting foreigners and members of the Haitian diaspora.

In addition, material donations act as a sign of good faith. In sending materials to the Justinien, Konbit Sante members prove they understand that it is dangerous and unpleasant to reuse latex gloves for surgeries; that it is devastating for Haitian clinicians to watch their patients die because of a lack of resources; and that, without basic tools and materials, clinicians cannot be effective. Because these gifts are not intended to be recirculated and because they are visible throughout the hospital, they serve as a constant reminder of Konbit Sante's efforts to ame-liorate working conditions at the Justinien. By leaving their material gifts in the hospital space, the givers leave a presence that adds to a constantly circulating cohort of volunteers. International aid is present as a subject of conversations; as a matter of speculation; in the form of objects that are used, stored, and dis-carded; and as a phenomenon whose impacts are never completely transparent or accounted for. Marcel Mauss (1950) drew on the Maori term *hau* to describe what he called the "spirit" of the gift—the tie that binds givers and receivers even after the specific gifting transaction has been completed.

When I asked the Justinien's staff to describe Konbit Sante's activities, they almost always began by telling me that the organization regularly sent large shipments of medical supplies, materials, and equipment to the hospital. The containers—which are shipped from Maine to the port of Cap-Haïtien and transported into the hospital's main courtyard by truck—are a tangible marker of Konbit Sante's support for the hospital. Common items include boxes of donated medications, medical equipment, electrical and plumbing supplies, and furniture. While other organizations ship materials to the Justinien on an occa-sional basis, Konbit Sante's donations are more frequent and regular, generally arriving at least twice a year. These shipments garner particular enthusiasm in Maine, where volunteers gather to sort supplies and load them in a collective effort. Preparing these shipments has been the subject of newspaper articles in Portland and essays on Konbit Sante's website, which are nearly always published with an accompanying photograph of the volunteers loading the containers.

Over time, preparing, shipping, and unloading the containers has become easier for the organization to manage. Nate Nickerson described the first con-tainer to arrive at the hospital, which took several days to unload and attracted a large number of men (not all of them hospital employees) who unloaded the items from the container and then expected to be paid for their work.[11] Since it has become known that unloading Konbit Sante's containers is not remuner-ated work, Nickerson reports that few if any workers come to help unload them. Nonetheless, the process now takes much less time than it used to, as the hospi-tal's newly inaugurated depot is prepared to receive donated goods. Other mech-anisms for distributing donated goods have developed over time—for example, if items in the container have been specifically donated for a certain service, that service will generally send staff to retrieve the items and bring them to the proper location.

In addition to the containers, the depot is a highly visible site for Konbit Sante's interventions. The structure, built in 2007 by the government of Haiti (with funding from USAID), consists of a 1,500-square-foot storage space and a small office for the depot manager. Not long after the new depot was built,

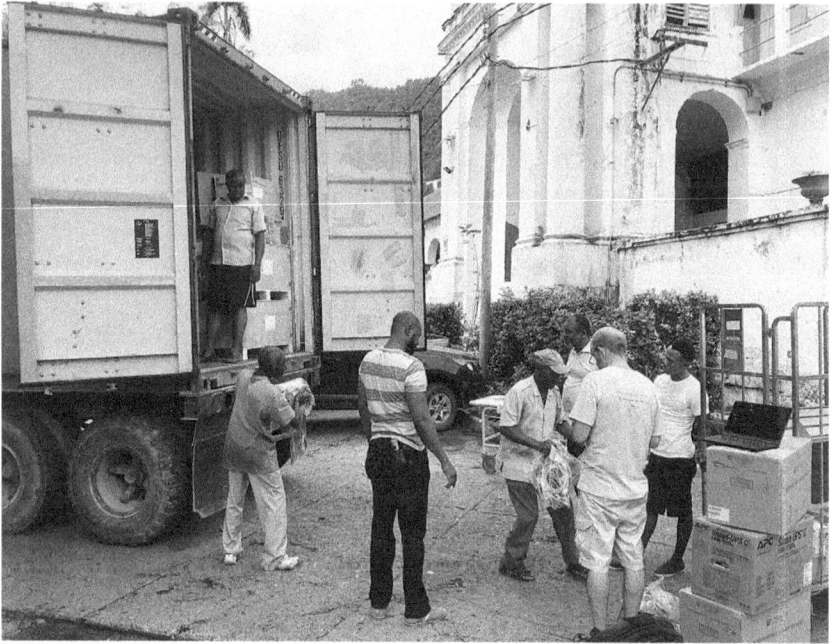

FIGURE 2.1.   Hôpital Universitaire Justinien and Konbit Sante employees unload a shipping container of medical supplies. August 2015. Photographer unknown. Image courtesy of Konbit Sante.

Konbit Sante equipped it with donated metal shelving units and hired a manager to be responsible for organizing the material, keeping track of inventory, and approving requisitions from hospital staff for needed supplies and medications. The hospital staff and Konbit Sante members describe the previous depot in unflattering terms: items were stored in disorganized heaps in a small room, it was never clear who had the key, and requests for materials were often unfulfilled. There appeared to be no oversight in terms of what came in or out of the depot, and many items were discarded after reaching their expiration date or sustaining physical damage from the conditions in which they were stored.

While the new depot was universally described as an improvement compared to the previous system, problems persist. Medical staff members complain that the items they need are not always available and that the depot's nonmedical personnel are not familiar with specialized pharmaceuticals or equipment and do not dispense them if they are requested by another name or brand. Some complain that the requisition process is too lengthy (a designated member of each service's staff is supposed to fill out a requisition form, drop it off at the depot, and return to retrieve the requested items). Certain members of the hospital's staff, particularly those in more senior medical positions, have taken to hoarding stocks of supplies in their own departments for greater autonomy.

Nevertheless, there is a regular stream of supplies in and out of the depot, and the hospital's administrative staff told me that the likelihood of attracting donations has increased tremendously now that they have a secure and controlled space for storing them. During my field research, the frequency of container donations did appear to increase significantly, and at times the depot manager was at a loss for where to store the increasing amount of donated supplies. In cases where it seemed as though medications and materials would expire before being used at the Justinien, the depot manager would contact clinics and hospitals in the surrounding area to distribute the excess. This informal arrangement highlights the importance of interpersonal networks for resource distribution in Haiti and exemplifies a situation in which individuals such as the depot manager could be accused of favoritism and of pilfering resources or diverting donations. The manager herself often told me that she experienced a great deal of pressure from others due to her position, but would not elaborate when I asked her for clarification.

Despite the limited emphasis their organization officially accords the provision of material goods and supplies, I was struck by Konbit Sante members' enthusiasm for and involvement with the containers and the depot while volunteers were in Haiti. American volunteers would often spend time in the depot when they were not occupied by meetings, training sessions, or site visits. They often expressed to me that working with supplies gave them "something concrete to do," and at the end of a sometimes frustrating day involving inconclusive meetings, delayed appointments, or various logistical obstacles, it was not uncommon to hear volunteers make comments such as, "Well, at least we got those boxes of medications sorted." Activities related to material aid could involve sorting newly arrived donations, classifying or rearranging stock on the shelves, moving items to ancillary storage spaces, or just tidying up.[12] I experienced this appeal firsthand, and found myself wandering to the depot during quieter times during my research, wanting to see what had been donated by which organizations, chatting with the depot staff, and observing how they were developing systems for organizing and distributing materials.

Various factors help explain this persistent interest in tangible forms of aid. Like many other foreigners, American members of Konbit Sante (particularly on their first visits to Haiti) were struck by the lack of physical resources at the Justinien and at other health care establishments. Many would make comparisons to conditions in the hospitals and clinics where they worked in the United States—scarcity and resourcefulness in Haiti to abundance and waste in their own workplaces. Konbit Sante volunteers spoke extensively and emotionally about the scarcity and lack of diversity of medications, medical materials, and medical equipment, often naming specific items that were absent ("They don't even have a refrigerator for medications that need to be kept at lower temperatures!") or out-of-date by their standards ("We used to use that kind of autoclave when I started working thirty years ago, but they're obsolete in Maine now!"). While the volunteers recognized and praised the Haitian medical staff's ingenuity and careful management in a context of limited resources, all the parties involved identified the latter as a major obstacle to providing high-quality medical services.

Another factor that made material forms of aid particularly seductive to North American volunteers was that much of the work related to material donations did not require Creole- or French-language skills or extensive negotiation. As opposed to meetings where personal contacts were often mediated through translators and painfully slow, Konbit Sante members could interact with material goods alongside non–English-speaking HUJ employees using nonverbal communication or without communicating at all. The supposedly redemptive qualities of physical labor are highlighted by the many aid groups that organize trips to Haiti and elsewhere for North Americans to build homes, paint schools, or renovate churches. While often described in glowing terms by the volunteer participants, these encounters do little to provide employment to Haitian carpenters, masons, or laborers. This model of aid is very different from the one formally promoted by Konbit Sante, but an enthusiasm for concrete interventions involving physical labor is nevertheless present among members of the group.

Those Konbit Sante volunteers and staff who had greater experience in Haiti, however, especially those who had assumed leadership positions in the organization, more often commented on resource scarcity as a systemic problem involving prioritization, organization, and distribution. In this discourse, they echoed the commonly heard refrain among Haitians that Haiti is rich but that its wealth has not been utilized or distributed in a just fashion. In contrast, however, members of Konbit Sante were more likely to talk about "weak systems" or "structural problems" than were Haitian hospital employees, who more often attributed resource scarcity to specific human failings such as incompetence, greed, lack of *konsyans* (conscience or awareness), or *mechanste* (meanness). Among members of other foreign aid groups, it was common to hear complaints about "corruption" in Haiti, particularly in terms of the Haitian state, even though those making the accusations often had had no experience with government workers or structures. Talk of corruption was not prominent among Konbit Sante members, who were much more likely to emphasize the challenges and constraints faced by employees in Haiti's public sector.

Material donations were usually the first of Konbit Sante's interventions to be mentioned by Haitian informants in their descriptions of the group's activities. This type of aid was particularly visible because containers entered the hospital through its main gates before being placed in the central courtyard for unloading. In addition, donated materials, equipment, and furniture often appeared throughout the hospital and frequently bore labels from donor institutions in Maine. Depot staff often wrote "HUJ/Konbit Sante" or simply "K.S." on items such as chairs or shelves in black permanent marker, which they hoped would deter potential thieves. Many of Konbit Sante's other activities (such as meetings, training sessions, and administrative work) took place behind closed doors, either in the group's small office on the hospital grounds or in other closed offices. While residents in pediatrics and internal medicine were aware that their physician supervisors were paid by Konbit Sante, they were not aware of the specific arrangements. Because Konbit Sante members interact primarily with upper-level staff at the Justinien, the only contact that most of the hospital's personnel would have with the organization would be through donated goods.

The tangible dimension of gifts such as bandages, pharmaceuticals, crutches, chairs, and surgical instruments confers a specific advantage to aid interventions, according to many hospital employees. Tangible objects with an immediate purpose are less ambiguous in function than cash and more apparent in presence than training or procedures. The flexibility and mutability of cash allow it to be used for unexpected expenses or redirected in cases of surplus but also make it easier for the donation to "take the wrong path" (*faire fausse route*), as my informants frequently observed. The notion of a "wrong path" for a donation implies the existence of a correct path: that aid has a singular and appropriate destination. In the discourse of my Haitian informants, monetary aid is particularly unlikely to make it down this path. In their words, "The people who need help the most don't receive it." The evidence for this is all around them—sick children, families living in squalor, and beggars in the street are all evidence of aid that failed to reach the appropriate recipients.[13] While noncash items could be sold or exchanged illicitly, the additional procedure this would require and the increased chances that the transaction would be exposed made donations of materials, equipment, and supplies among the "safest."

Some of the group's North American staff and volunteers were aware of the prominence that material donations had in the eyes of the Justinien's staff and at times found this to be disconcerting. Unlike other organizations for which material medical aid is a primary activity and reason for existence,[14] Konbit Sante always lists activities related to donations and supplies low on its descriptions of programs, after activities such as training, administrative support, infrastructure development, and research. The group presents these activities within the larger framework of capacity building, a concept that emerged within the UN system and financial institutions such as the World Bank and the IMF in the late twentieth century. Capacity building minimizes the provision of material goods, and instead emphasizes restructuring organizations and value systems and developing human resources (Wubneh 2003). Not only do Konbit Sante members feel that attention to material donations may distract from their primary objectives and strategies but they are also concerned that tangible forms of aid to one of the hospital's services will be noticed by members of other services and attract even more solicitations or resentment in cases of refusal. The members of Konbit Sante are accustomed to regular and repeated solicitations for diverse forms of aid from individuals, groups, and institutions. Nickerson commented to me that it sometimes felt like he spent most of his time in Haiti fielding and turning down requests for material support. Despite their frequency and ubiquity, solicitations of aid remain unsettling for members of Konbit Sante, and many describe them as the most difficult aspect of spending time in Haiti. At the same time, it seems unlikely that the organization will stop sending material donations to Haiti. Maine-based staff and volunteers witness the material constraints that make biomedical practice challenging in Haiti, and they have a real desire to improve the conditions in which Haitian health professionals treat their patients. In addition, the material supplies that Konbit Sante has sent act as a foot in the door, not only by creating an ongoing tie between donors and recipients but also by facilitating other types of interventions, including trainings, changes in management, and administrative projects, which are more sensitive and politically charged in nature.

Giving, Receiving, and Reciprocating

Organizing medical aid to Haiti in the form of material donations fits with a deficit model, where recipient groups are defined solely according to what they are perceived to be lacking, and interventions are structured in order to transfer resources from areas of wealth and surplus to areas deemed deficient. This dynamic exists elsewhere: Ramah McKay (2018) describes how the work of health volunteers in Mozambique "transformed the 'needs of the community' into a potential resource through the intervention of transnational donors" (61). In this case, resources included tangible objects such as bicycles, soap, buckets, bandages, and other materials. While McKay was initially frustrated by volunteers' preoccupation with obtaining material resources (as opposed to focusing on caring for vulnerable members of the community), she came to realize that this preoccupation and care were complementary rather than contradictory. The deficit model is not the exclusive terrain of foreigners working in Haiti; it is also prominent in Haitians' discourses, which often negate existing resources ("Sa se pa yon lopital" [This isn't a hospital], "Nou pa gen wout" [we don't have roads]). This practice, which I term *rhetorical negation*, also serves to make a case that aid is truly needed and, as I described in the previous chapter, impedes the coordination of aid efforts. This rhetorical negation also resonates with a widespread sense of irony in Haiti: I frequently heard Haitians point out that, despite its widespread poverty, Haiti is not really poor; rather, the country's riches (in the form of minerals, natural beauty, agricultural resources, and a youthful population) are not being utilized to benefit the country's citizens. This observation poses a critique to the deficit model, and the importation of material aid to Haiti becomes an aggressive and poisonous gift, as it is not *truly* needed, but rather works to keep Haiti in a perpetual state of dependence and underdevelopment.

Even if Konbit Sante's interventions in the Justinien did not include any material components, they could still be classified as gifts according to Mauss's classic definition, which includes intangible services as well as goods (1950, 3–7). Because goods and tangible objects have eclipsed conceptions of services as gifts not only in academic literature but also in popular understandings of the term, I suspect that most members of Konbit Sante would not think of trainings for health agents or analyses of the hospital's water supply as gifts. Gift giving also creates categories of givers and receivers, which contradicts the group's emphasis on partners and colleagues. Nevertheless, gift language permeated Konbit Sante's descriptions of even the most intangible interventions: "to *give* them the tools to be self-sufficient," "to *provide* support for hospital staff," "to *contribute* to infrastructure in Haiti." The equipment, supplies, and pharmaceuticals sent to the Justinien are even more obviously classifiable as gifts by both Americans and Haitians, although the word *gift* was almost never used: *donation* was the term of choice.[15]

Mauss famously categorized giving, reciprocating, and receiving as obligations and described situations in various societies where these obligations help ensure harmonious social relations within and between groups. All three obligations are described, enforced, and contested differently depending on the models of giving and values present in a given society. Elsewhere, I have described the tensions related to giving that emerge out of two distinct (but increasingly overlapping) rhetorics involved in the provision of care to Haitians at a Dominican border hospital (Minn 2010). In humanitarian rhetoric, aid results from a donor's will to give and can be stopped or rescinded at any time. In human rights rhetoric, providers are obligated to aid a patient in order to protect the latter's human right to health; withholding aid could constitute a human rights violation. Although Konbit Sante members promote the idea that health is a human right (this position is the first item on the group's "About Us" page on its website), they do not make an explicit link between Haitians' right to health and their own obligation to provide health services. Their choice of Haiti as a site of intervention did not stem from a prior relationship or a sense of obligation based on kinship or nationality, as is the case for many Haitian diaspora groups. Rather, they chose Haiti because of its proximity to Maine (initial efforts to work in Africa were abandoned because of distance) and because it was there that they saw "the greatest need." I never heard the group's members speak about their activities in Haiti in terms of an obligation to give; however, they did use the term *give back*, an expression that implies reciprocity.

Konbit Sante members spoke about an obligation to receive that became apparent not long after the group began intervening in Haiti. This involved group members offering a resource or service, which would be accepted, often eagerly, by hospital staff. On subsequent visits, however, group members would notice that the intended resource or service was not being used, and in the case of physical objects was often collecting dust in a storage space. This created speculation among American staff and volunteers about the reasons for what appeared to be a blanket acceptance of all offers. One told me, "Even though they said that this was going to be helpful, it's in the discard pile. And we'd love to figure out a way to work with our Haitian colleagues to get to a more candid appraisal of things that they really don't want." When I asked him why he thought such an appraisal was difficult to obtain, he replied, "It's very hard to say no to your uncle, to your rich uncle that brings you all this stuff. . . . Maybe he won't bring you anything [the next time]." Another volunteer used the phrase, "You don't bite the hand that feeds you," confirming that some North American informants were aware of the power differential that exists between donors and recipients in such transactions. While both North American and Haitian informants pointed to some pragmatic reasons why aid was seldom refused (the aid might not be useful at the time of donation, but a corresponding need could arise with time; an item that was not particularly useful could be disassembled for parts and materials), a key factor identified by all informants was that a refusal could decrease the likelihood of future offers of aid, either because the donor might assume that the recipient was not, in fact, needy, or because once an alternate recipient had been identified for the rejected gift, the channel of aid might be diverted away from the original recipient. While they usually did not make these reflections explicit in their interactions with each other, many of the Konbit Sante members and all the hospital staff I spoke with about these issues recognized that the obligation to receive was central to perpetuating gift relations.

Finally, the obligation to reciprocate is particularly contentious in the aid I studied. At first glance, Konbit Sante's interventions in Haiti, like those of many international medical aid groups, can be interpreted as unreciprocated gifts. Whether the aid takes the form of material donations or transfers of expertise or capacity-building activities, the most obvious flow of goods and resources is from wealthy countries to Haiti, with no obvious reciprocal countergift. It would be difficult to conceive of the Haitian government or Haitian organizations sending medicine or supplies to the United States, Canada, or France. That being said, reciprocity should not be dismissed as irrelevant to this context, as it was a central if not always explicit theme in many of the discourses, actions, and relationships I observed among both Haitian and non-Haitian participants in international medical aid.

One manifestation of reciprocity appeared in the discourses of Konbit Sante volunteers and other North American medical aid volunteers, who said that their activities in Haiti were a form of "giving back." This expression was used by individuals who may never have been to Haiti and often had no prior relationship with Haitian people. When asked to elaborate what they meant, informants told me that they felt that they had received a great deal in terms of opportunities, resources, and good fortune, which let them enjoy a high quality of life. They understood their activities in Haiti to be an appropriate response for someone in their position. By framing these activities as "giving back," the volunteers did not assume that impoverished Haitians were the specific source of their own successes and comfortable lifestyles; rather, they felt that they had been blessed or favored by a nonspecific force such as "fate" or "being born in the right place at the right time." Work in Haiti reciprocated these gifts of ambiguous origin to people who desperately needed the available countergift. While the volunteers could and did give back through various activities in their home state of Maine, work in Haiti is particularly satisfying for Konbit Sante volunteers because of the enormous needs they identify there.

Another commonly used phrase that suggested the salience of reciprocity among Konbit Sante members and other North American aid workers was "I get so much more out of doing this than I give." This phrase was most often used when responding to praise by observers for the speakers' work in Haiti. When they were asked what it was they "got" out of doing aid work, responses generally revolved around the satisfaction of being able to help others and "accomplish something." One described the feeling associated with working in Haiti as a drug: "Once you start, you get hooked!" Many appreciated the contact they shared with Haitian colleagues and the relationships they had built with them over time. Some mentioned enjoying the opportunity of seeing another country and culture, although witnessing poverty and pathology for Haiti also represented a source of pain and negative emotions. In many cases, however, it seemed that saying they got more than they received from working in Haiti was a way of deflecting admiration. Whether because of social conventions that require modesty from the doers of good deeds or because of a discomfort with what might seem like excessive adulation for an activity that has become a routine part of their lives, bringing reciprocity into play allows aid workers to avoid being characterized as *selfless* and *altruistic* (terms most aid workers I met did not identify with) or as the magnanimous distributors of nonreciprocal gifts, complete with the discrepancies in power that accompanies this role.

A final manifestation of reciprocity in the work of Konbit Sante and other international groups working in Haiti involves the emigration of Haitian medical staff to the countries where the bulk of the aid originates, specifically the United States, Canada, and France. The experiences and relationships these health professionals have with international aid bodies is the subject of the following chapter. I will simply mention here that these professionals' emigration to aid-sending countries could be framed as a form of reciprocity, in which Haitian professionals return the gift of training and employment in Haiti with emigration to and service in the sending country. I was frequently told that employment with an international organization often acts as a stepping-stone toward emigration. This was the case for Dr. Gilles, who was Konbit Sante's in-country program manager when I arrived in Haiti. A Haitian-trained physician, he also had an MPH from an American university and spoke fairly fluent English. After working for Konbit Sante for several years, he emigrated with his family to Canada, where he found a job doing manual labor in a food-packing plant.[16]

While this type of emigration could be interpreted as reciprocity, it was never framed as such by any of my Haitian informants. Rather, emigration represented an opportunity for personal advancement, even if the gains of this advancement would ultimately be shared with family members and other members of one's network. When individuals involved in medical aid spoke of Haitian health professionals' obligations to work in a particular location, it was always in reference to Haiti and often to the specific locality the professional hailed from. I assume that Haitian health professionals themselves did not feel an obligation to reciprocate to donor countries because these countries are too wealthy to warrant a countergift, or because they conceive of aid from donor countries not as constituting a gift but, rather, as contributing to Haiti's worsening social, political, and economic climate.

In this chapter, I have focused on the work of a small, secular North American medical organization in Haiti. By choosing not to carry out clinical interventions, Konbit Sante has relinquished one of the most powerful images of humanitarian activity in favor of a more administrative and systemic model of international medical intervention. Nevertheless, the group's members continue to face many of the same tensions and struggles as organizations working within more established and conventional models of medical aid. Most of the preceding discussion and analysis of Konbit Sante, its activities, and the gift relations the group engenders and negotiates have been informed by the perspectives and data collected from the group's American staff and volunteers. In the following chapter, I will discuss the Haitian medical staff's views of the international interventions they encounter as part of their daily activities. I will also return to the theme of obligation, as young Haitian physicians debate their departures for the very countries that send them aid in various forms.

BETWEEN A FUND AND A HARD PLACE

On a warm spring evening, I sat with a Haitian physician in the dusty courtyard of a small rural hospital as he met with a dozen men and women who worked there as cleaners, janitors, and maintenance workers. The physician, a middle-aged man with a fatherly demeanor, had been hired by the American NGO that ran the hospital in partnership with the Haitian Ministry of Health to determine which staff members were in fact employees of the establishment. As in many Haitian public hospitals, not all of the people who worked there were on the government's payroll; some had taken over positions left vacant when relatives had died.[1] Others had been hired for short-term contracts years ago and continued working through informal arrangements with the hospital's director. The visiting doctor's questions about how many years they had worked at the hospital and their specific functions were met with evasive answers and elaborate descriptions of economic difficulties, struggling households, and dependent families. Unable to distinguish official from de facto employees, he exclaimed in frustration: "Look—everyone's got someone pushing in their back!"

This image of being pushed in the back comes to life in Haiti during elections, school registrations, and distributions of various kinds. When the stakes are high and outcomes uncertain, people will stand crammed against each other so that any movement at the back of the line is felt by those in the front, causing more stress and anxiety in an already tense situation. By using the pushing metaphor, the physician signaled to the hospital staff that, while he understood their financial obligations and the importance of their meager salaries in fulfilling them, he was also experiencing pressures, specifically from the foreign organization who had hired him to clarify the ambiguities and confusion regarding the hospital's staffing.

In this chapter, I analyze the situation of Haitian health professionals. Those who work closely with international interventions often find themselves in a situation that I describe as being between a fund and a hard place. The "fund" refers to the diverse resources (including money, equipment and supplies, medical services, and employment opportunities) that these professionals, through their involvement with international medical aid, are expected to disburse and channel to patients and others in need; they also represent possibilities for their own professional and personal advancement. The "hard place" refers to the plight of the majority of Haitians, whose grueling lives are marked by poverty, hard labor, poor health, and an uncertain future. The physicians, nurses, and other health professionals—who are increasingly hired to implement, manage, and disburse international medical aid—are forced to negotiate a range of conflicting pressures that originate both in front of and behind them in the metaphorical line.

Haitian health professionals' involvement with such aid is varied. Some are involved to a significant degree, such as clinical personnel hired by foreign NGOs, medical students and residents receiving training in foreign-sponsored medical school and residency programs, and the administrators and personnel of large international interventions. Lesser degrees of involvement may include fitting a patient for a pair of crutches donated by an international organization, getting a week off work because a foreign surgical team has taken over the operating room, or speculating from a distance about the origin of the foreigners taking pictures of infants in a hospital's neonatal unit.

The context for the meeting I described at the beginning of this chapter is a revealing example of several forces at play in international medical aid in Haiti. The hospital, like many public health establishments throughout the country, had been understaffed and underresourced for years. With the death of its long-term medical director in 2002, it had fallen into severe disrepair, with no electricity, running water, or regular shipments of pharmaceuticals and basic medical supplies. It was the only government-run health establishment for a population of eighty thousand people. In 2006 the leaders of an American-based NGO that had been operating a small clinic in the area approached the Haitian Ministry of Health with the goal of forming a partnership to revitalize the hospital. The ministry would renovate the building and provide salaries for certain members of the hospital's staff; the NGO would move its clinical activities from its small dispensary to the larger hospital while continuing to raise funds and seek out grants. The doctor who used the pushing metaphor during the meeting was hired as a consultant by the NGO to help clarify the hospital's staffing and operations. He was recruited in part because of his experience working with another American

NGO; he eventually left both organizations because he felt that his remuneration was insufficient.

Two trends have been particularly significant in shaping the work and lives of Haiti's health professionals in recent decades. The first has been the increase in international institutions, projects, and campaigns that train and hire Haitian employees for a wide range of positions, including administrators, physicians, nurses, laboratory and other technicians, and community health workers. These initiatives also hire an important number of support and ancillary staff, such as cleaning and maintenance staff, drivers, and others. This development is part of an increasing emphasis on the role of local human resources in health, visible in the World Health Organization's 2006 *World Health Report*, which states that "at the heart of each and every health system, the workforce is central to advancing health." This report, like many others, identified a lack in health care workers that has a negative impact on populations' health. Health care workers are not just responsible for carrying out technical procedures and dispensing health services; they "are the personification of a system's core values—they heal and care for people, ease pain and suffering, prevent disease and mitigate risk—the human link that connects knowledge to health action" (WHO 2006). Whereas earlier international health initiatives relied more on expatriate health workers (and certain programs continue to do so), it is increasingly common for foreign organizations and agencies not only to hire but also to train local health workers.

The second trend is the emigration of health workers from Haiti, particularly to the United States, the Dominican Republic, Canada, and France. Health workers were prominent among the professionals who emigrated from Haiti in the 1960s (Glick Schiller and Fouron 2001; Fagen 2009), and while the percentage of professionals among Haitian emigrants decreased significantly in subsequent decades (Portes and Grosfoguel 1994, 58), a report by the World Bank estimated that 83.6 percent of tertiary-educated individuals in Haiti were emigrating in 2000 (World Bank 2011). The same report cites a study that found that over 35 percent of Haitian physicians emigrate annually (Bhargavan, Docquier, and Moullan 2011, 176).

While these two trends are not necessarily causally related, my informants drew explicit links between the two. Like Dr. Célestin in the introduction to this book, Haitian health professionals often consider working for an international NGO to be a stepping-stone for emigration—in terms of the experience, language skills, and contacts that are often gained through such work, as well as the possibility to amass the capital needed to leave Haiti since NGOs generally pay higher salaries than those offered by the Haitian government.

After a brief overview of Haitian health workers' historical contact with foreign medical interventions, I discuss the situation of a specific group of health workers: the medical residents at the Justinien. In addition to providing basic demographic information about the residents, I describe a labor strike that took place during my research in order to highlight how medical professionals in Haiti interpret and respond to the challenges they face. I go on to describe some features of the residents' contact with international medical aid bodies. These features, as well as the residents' reflections on aid, illustrate how Haitian medical professionals view, critique, and work with and against international interventions. I then discuss the phenomenon most often referred to as "brain drain," and the links between international medical aid and the emigration of Haitian health professionals. I close this chapter by discussing the theme of obligation and its multiple meanings in this context.

Historical Antecedents

Haitians have been providing health care in the context of foreign intervention, occupation, and domination for centuries. In tracing the historical roots of Haitian practitioners' involvement in international medical work, my goal is not to equate an eighteenth-century enslaved *hospitalière* with a twenty-first-century nurse employed by a Canadian NGO. Such a comparison might serve as a provocative commentary on power relations and autonomy in the world of contemporary international aid, but also risks banalizing the extreme and horrific nature of chattel slavery in colonial Saint-Domingue, minimizing the significance and impact of the Haitian Revolution, and suggesting equivalence between very different historical and sociopolitical contexts. Rather, my goal is to trace the occupational heritage of contemporary Haitian health workers and identify points of similarity or divergence with previous forms of healing on the island. Doing so brings into relief the fact that since the colonial era, medical practice in Saint-Domingue and Haiti has been closely intertwined with political and economic forces in other countries, particularly those originating in France and the United States.

Although hospitals in eighteenth-century Saint-Domingue included military hospitals—*hôtels-Dieu* (for strictly medical care) and *hôpitaux généraux* (that served to confine beggars and other socially undesirable individuals)—the predominant medical establishment during the French colonial period was the plantation hospital (Brodwin 1996, 29–32). These establishments developed along with the rise of the sugar industry in the Caribbean, and while free and European doctors were sometimes summoned to treat certain ailments among slaves, plantation hospitals were principally staffed with slaves. These individuals found themselves in the aberrant position of being forced to provide care for fellow slaves whose labor enriched the owners of the patients and the healers themselves. The "enslaved healers" of Saint-Domingue included *hospitalières* (women in charge of plantation hospitals), *infirmières* (nurses or hospital aides), *accoucheuses* (midwives), and herbalists and spiritual healers (Weaver 2006, 42–58). Karol Weaver states that plantation medicine was extremely lucrative for European surgeons, and claims that many young surgeons traveled to Saint-Domingue from France in search of riches (46–47). This phenomenon may be a direct antecedent of the contemporary belief, widespread among Haitian physicians, that foreign and diaspora health workers are attracted to medical work in Haiti for monetary gain.

Not surprisingly, relationships between masters and enslaved healers were fraught on several levels. One of the most contentious aspects of healers' work in colonial Saint-Domingue was the practice of abortion or infanticide. Enslaved mothers and midwives were frequently suspected of using herbal treatments or other means to induce abortion, cause infantile tetanus, or kill newborns outright. Whites in the colony suspected that this was done to keep infants from becoming slaves. Enslaved healers were also suspected of using their knowledge of herbal remedies to poison whites; verified cases of poisoning from historical accounts confirm that this was a well-founded fear. Other practices, such as providing hospitalization for malingering slaves and pilfering resources from plantation owners, illustrate the complex array of choices and moral quandaries that were a part of daily life for enslaved healers during the colonial period (Weaver 2006).

In the years following the revolution, plantation hospitals persisted, as did military hospitals and hospices operated by Catholic orders. Medical education for Haitians was limited, however, with only sporadic and short-lived efforts to train Haitian health workers in the early nineteenth-century. The national medical school began granting degrees in 1870, and in the decades that followed, hospitals founded by private citizens opened in major cities throughout Haiti (Brodwin 1996, 44–45, 48). The Justinien is an example of an institution that was established during this period.

The US Marine occupation of Haiti, which lasted from 1915 to 1934, radically transformed medical practice throughout the country. The occupation is generally viewed critically by contemporary scholars, who decry its racist underpinnings, the physical brutality of its personnel, the economic exploitation it facilitated, and its centralization of power in Port-au-Prince. Among the few positive legacies of the US occupation were the construction of hospitals throughout the country, the development of bureaucratic and administrative structures for a public health system, and the introduction of modern nursing to Haiti. Dr. Ary Bordes, the preeminent historian of medicine in Haiti, gave a detailed account of medicine and public health during the American occupation (Bordes 1992).

He traced the early medical efforts by the occupying forces, which centered first on medical services for American soldiers and the newly formed Gendarmerie d'Haïti (Haitian Constabulary), and the creation of the Service nationale d'hygiène publique (National Public Hygiene Service), which would eventually become the country's Ministry of Health. This service focused on public hygiene and sanitation, the treatment and control of infectious diseases, and the development of health facilities. Bordes argues that the service's focus on urban sanitation and health also entailed a neglect of rural Haitians, which represented 95 percent of Haiti's population during the American occupation (1992, 95–96).

In the early twentieth century, there were fewer than one hundred physicians in the entire country, most of them working in Port-au-Prince. As a reflection of the Francophile intellectual and social trends of the era among the Haitian middle and upper classes (Valdman 1984), many had completed basic or supplementary medical studies in France, but few had studied in the United States, a destination with far less appeal (Bordes 1992, 34). In the twentieth century, however, Marcus Cueto describes the "increasing process of 'Americanization' and a corresponding decline of European influence, especially French influence, in Latin American medicine and medical sciences more broadly" (Cueto 1994a, xv). Regarding the Rockefeller Foundation's activities in Latin America, Cueto writes,

> Shortly after their creation in the early twentieth century, American philanthropies began to export to less-developed countries institutional models for the organization of knowledge, under the assumption that the giver knew what was good for the receiver. This assumption reflected the institutions' perceptions of isolated elements of foreign cultures, and their comparisons of these perceptions with social, cultural, and scientific developments in the United States. . . . There were constant references to the role that German-trained U.S. students played in the modernization of medical education and research in the United States. Foundation officers became sincerely convinced that the RF would play the same role in Latin American science and medicine that Germany had played in the reorganization of U.S. science. RF officials proceeded from a main assumption—that the most-advanced Latin American institutions and societies could replicate the development of their counterparts in the United States. (Cueto 1994b, 1, 13–14)

In his subsequent volume tracing the history of medicine in Haiti following the American occupation, Bordes frames his findings in a discussion of Haitian society more broadly, arguing that the hierarchies and divisions that marked the colonial period remained in large part intact during the middle of the twentieth century, but was also marked by the emergence of a Black middle class in the

1940s, a group that he claimed would join the mulatto elite in oppressing the rural masses (Bordes 1997, 24). He also traces the earliest permanent migrations of Haitian health professionals to the metropolitan areas in the northeastern United States and Canada and in lesser numbers to Liberia and Venezuela. (This flow would increase in the 1960s as health professionals fled the repressive Duvalier dictatorship.)

While limited in comparison with the present-day situation, the scope and diversity of international interventions increased during the middle of the twentieth century. Bordes traces the implementation of a number of projects by different international actors: the construction of clinics, hospitals, latrines, and other infrastructure projects (implemented by the Rockefeller-funded American Sanitary Mission); yaws eradication and health worker training (by the Inter-American Cooperation Service of Public Health); and insect control, research, training, and laboratory support (by the Pan-American Health Bureau). He also describes the activities of various UN agencies (UNESCO, UNICEF, FAO, WHO, etc.) and the early implantation of NGOs such as CARE. Bordes identifies yaws eradication as the greatest medical success in the country during this period. The most famous medical professional involved in this campaign was none other than the future dictator François "Papa Doc" Duvalier. The historian's assessment of international aid in the second half of the twentieth century is bleak: "In the decades to come, the role of international assistance would increase and the country would become increasingly dependent on foreign aid, without ever being able to resolve its health problems. Our leaders should be aware of the role, reach, limits and use of external assistance if they wish to avoid being disillusioned by the promises of international diplomacy and the mirages of international organizations" (Bordes 1997, 214–15).

Little has been written about health and international intervention during the Duvalier dictatorship. In more general terms, scholars have addressed the suspension and renewal of American aid to the Haitian government under the Kennedy and Nixon administrations, respectively, and the increasing reliance on NGOs to support foreign programs in health, agriculture, and education during this period (Buss 2008, 70–71). This period also saw an increase in French Canadian Catholic missionaries in Haiti, who had begun to travel to Haiti during the presidency of Élie Lescot in the 1940s. Many of these nuns, brothers, and priests were involved in health interventions through hospitals, clinics, and dispensaries run by their religious orders (Mills 2016). During the 1960s, Haiti was the destination of 27 percent of Catholic missionaries leaving Quebec, and in 2004, four hundred remained in the country (Icart 2004). These missionaries were known for spending relatively long periods in the country (missions frequently lasted several decades), which allowed them to gain fluency in Haitian Creole and become deeply knowledgeable about local social and community structures. Grace Sanders (2010) suggests that relationships between Canadian missionaries and Haitians were extremely hierarchical, a pattern that shifted as the missionaries aged, creating a need to rely increasingly on younger Haitian clergy and medical professionals.

Haitian Health Care Workers Today

Demographic information in Haiti, including data about employment and occupations, is extremely difficult to obtain. Censuses are conducted only sporadically, and many demographic estimates are based on imprecise and dated calculations. The population of the city of Cap-Haïtien, for example, has been estimated to be anywhere from 100,000 (Oxfam 2010) to 800,000 (Foreign and Commonwealth Office 2009). Estimates of the number of health care workers have largely been based on conjecture or simply absent. In 2007 the Projet d'Appui au renforcement des capacités en gestion de la santé en Haïti (PARC), a project based at the University of Montreal's International Health Unit, partnered with the Haitian Ministry of Health to conduct a nationwide census of health care workers. In addition to collecting basic demographic information, the census also recorded the occupational specialty and type of employer for each health professional. The census also collected information about medical education and training in Haiti, and about the emigration of recent graduates. The scope and detail of this census, which relied on a team of over sixty individuals, are impressive, and provide valuable information on the human resources and staffing of health establishments in Haiti. The motivation behind the census was to "equip [MSPP] to develop and put into place policies for human resources that are adapted to the needs of the health system" (Dubois 2004, 5). The census offers one of the few comprehensive and reliable sources of data on Haitian health care workers.

The census reports that there were 2.61 health workers per 1,000 individuals, one of the lowest rates in the world. It also states that 40 percent of the 24,278 health care workers were support, administrative, or logistics staff, a higher percentage than in most other countries. Only 31 percent of health care workers had university-level training, and only 27 percent had a professional status that qualified them to provide services autonomously (physician, nurse, midwife, dentist, pharmacist, etc.). In terms of ratios in the professional categories, approximately 10 percent of health workers were physicians, who were slightly outnumbered by nurses and midwives (13 percent). Clinical aides and auxiliary nurses represented 27 percent of all health workers.

According to the census, Haiti's ratio of physicians and nurses is only .59 per 1,000 individuals, which is far below the WHO's recommended rate of 2.5, the rate the organization claims is needed to provide basic vaccines for 80 percent of the population and safe childbirth for 80 percent of pregnant women (Dubois 2004, 11). The PARC census also found that public institutions have the highest percentage of support, logistical, and administrative staff, a rate of 42 percent compared to a rate of 28 percent in private establishments. However, private establishments employ a much higher rate of medical technicians than public establishments, owing in part to the prevalence of private laboratories and the paucity of laboratory resources in most public clinics and hospitals.

Other findings include that 66 percent of health care workers are under the age of forty-five, and that nearly half of them (46 percent) work in Port-au-Prince and its surrounding areas. The census found that a minority of health care workers (18 percent) worked in primary care facilities such as dispensaries and health centers, which are often the only medical establishments that are easily accessible for rural populations. Almost half of health care workers are employed in hospitals (generally located in urban areas), private clinics, and MSPP offices, and, in such settings, are not accessible for impoverished and/or rural patients.

Haitian health care professionals have not been the subject of significant attention by social scientists. When mentioned by medical anthropologists, they often appear as secondary figures, either as obstacles to satisfactory patient care, or less frequently, as heroic supporters of medicine for all. In Catherine Maternowska's (2006) thorough analysis of a family planning clinic in the Port-au-Prince slum of Cité Soleil, physicians represent "a small slice of Haiti's privileged class" (75). During their extremely brief consultations with patients, they bark orders, dismiss medical and economic concerns, and are disconnected from the rest of the clinic staff (95). They are there to provide technical skills only, and work at the clinic "only for the extra cash" (95). Although Maternowska found that doctors and nurses analyze and understand the macrolevel forces that shape fertility and contraception use in Haiti, "the understanding of macro forces was distinctly removed from the micro situation in the clinic—or the community—and their analyses did not appear to inform their treatment or discussion of clients. Indeed, their analyses confirmed an enormous gap between insight and practice" (96). The author suggests that these tensions are systemic rather than individuals' failings by describing the clinic's director:

> When he formerly worked as a clinician, he would often joke with the clients and engage in their lives. Frequently he would go out of his way to help someone in need. He was a *dòk* [doctor] that everyone loved. As the

son of two farmers, he was one of the lucky (and few) brilliant students who actually made it into Haiti's state-managed medical school without ties to the upper classes. Years of working at this clinic and dealing with the rigorous demands of international agencies had slowly transformed this man from a humble, client-devoted doctor to a hard, urban bureaucrat who directed the clinic. (94)

While Maternowska acknowledges some of the institutional and structural constraints that health professionals face (resource scarcity, little credit or recognition for their efforts, boring and repetitive work), her account focuses on the ways they perpetuate and reinforce hierarchies and inequalities in Haitian society, to the detriment of their impoverished patients.

Paul Brodwin's (1996) description of nurses is similar—he describes a "code of deference," or "the mutual expectations and taken-for-granted rules which pattern unfolding activities," including provider-patient interactions in a rural Haitian dispensary. Nurses and nurse auxiliaries publicly criticize and shame patients in the dispensary's waiting room, using their cases as examples for other patients and as opportunities to deliver instructions on proper nutrition, the care of children, and other matters. Brodwin compares these interactions to those that take place in schools and courthouses: "social relations that are formal, authoritarian, and partially inscrutable to the petitioners below" (67). In rural areas such as the village where Brodwin conducted his research, physicians often do not have a permanent presence, but rather carry out rotations as part of their mandatory year of social service upon completing medical school, or as part of an arrangement through international NGOs to attend to patients in several clinics in a geographic area.

My findings complicate these analyses. It became apparent during my research with the medical residents at the Justinien that they do not originate from Haiti's elite in the way that physicians of previous generations did. Since the 1990s, many members of Haiti's wealthiest and most elite families have migrated abroad. Those who remain may send their children to private secondary schools in Port-au-Prince (including internationally accredited schools such as the Lycée Alexandre Dumas or the Union School, founded during the 1915–34 occupation for the children of US military families stationed in Haiti), and students from the wealthiest families generally attend university outside of Haiti. Students entering medical school in Haiti (which is an undergraduate degree) are much more likely to come from Haiti's small middle class, which is intimately connected to Haitian diasporic populations in North America. While spared the economic plight of Haiti's impoverished masses, these young physicians remain subject to significant instability and insecurity about their future prospects.

The Residents at the Justinien

During my research, there were fifty-four medical residents at the hospital, pursuing either three-year (pediatrics, obstetrics/gynecology, internal medicine, urology, family practice) or four-year (surgery, orthopedics, anesthesiology) specializations. I conducted in-depth interviews with fifty-two of the residents, using an open-ended questionnaire that focused on international interventions and the practice of medicine at the Justinien and in Haiti more broadly.[2] I chose to interview the medical residents for a number of reasons. Out of all of the hospital's medical staff, the residents spent the most time at the establishment. At any given moment, approximately thirty-five residents lived on the hospital's campus. The remainder lived with relatives or rented rooms in Cap-Haïtien, and others left periodically on rotations to other hospitals in Haiti. As residents were prohibited from seeing patients in private practice, they devoted all of their efforts to their work at the hospital. In this way, they were not only intimately familiar with the hospital's services and operation but also became a constant presence during my research, much more familiar than the attending physicians. Nurses were fairly consistent in attending their shifts, but these shifts were often quite short, and they, like the attending physicians, also worked in private practice and other sectors such as commerce and teaching, which reduced their presence and availability at the Justinien.

Medical education in Haiti follows a European model, in which students enter medical school after completing high school and taking an entrance exam. During the time of my research, there were four government-recognized medical schools in Haitian universities. These included the Université d'État d'Haïti, the state university with a graduating class of about one hundred medical students annually; Université Notre-Dame d'Haïti and Université Quisqueya, private universities with graduating classes of approximately fifty students each; and Université Lumière, a much smaller university with a graduating class of a dozen medical students.

With a single exception, the residents at the Justinien had all studied at Université Notre-Dame d'Haïti or Université Quisqueya, the two major private universities.[3] Residency positions at the capital's main public hospital, the Hôpital de l'Université d'État d'Haïti are reserved for graduates of the state university, an arrangement that greatly displeased many of the residents, who would rather have stayed in Port-au-Prince. (The residents complained that to enter the state university's medical school, one had to have personal contacts. Tuition at the state university is nominal when compared to the private universities; how the quality of education compares between establishments is a subject of intense debate.)

Looking at basic demographic indicators for the medical residents at the HUJ, several patterns emerged. About half of the residents were from Port-au-Prince, a quarter from Cap-Haïtien and its surrounding areas, and the remainder from other parts of Haiti, generally from cities and larger villages. Thirty-one of the residents were women, twenty-three were men, and they ranged in age from twenty-seven to thirty-six. Nearly all of them had attended private schools run by Catholic religious orders for their primary and secondary education. With the exception of the few elite international schools in Port-au-Prince, these Catholic schools are widely considered to provide the best education in Haiti. Asking about their parents' professions, I was surprised to find that only four had a parent who was a physician and only five had a parent who was a nurse. Instead, some of the residents' parents were professionals (primary school teachers, secretaries, lower-ranking government workers), while the majority worked in trades (commerce, food service, tailoring, and other occupations). I recall my surprise at meeting a woman who I assumed (because of her dress, demeanor, and speech) to be a resident's hired domestic employee, when in fact she was the physician's mother, and her primary occupation was small-scale commerce.[4] While I heard both state university-trained Haitian physicians and international health care workers claim that the graduates of private universities came from wealthier families who could afford higher tuition (approximately 700 USD at the time of my study), the residents at the Justinien denied this claim. From my interviews, however, I learned that nearly every resident had close relatives living abroad, including parents, aunts, uncles, and siblings. Given the importance of overseas remittances by migrants to household incomes in Haiti, it is likely that these residents' access to higher education was facilitated by contributions from relatives abroad. However, these contributions may not have been sufficient to enable the residents' own migration and education abroad, at least not at that point in their lives.

The residents occupy an interstitial position in professional hierarchies at the Justinien. As physicians, they have greater prestige and authority than most of the hospital's staff, including nurses, auxiliaries, interns, and almost all nonmedical personnel. However, as the youngest physicians, and because of the relative brevity of their presence at the hospital, they have little sway or decision-making power when compared to the attending physicians or senior members of the hospital's administration. Patients often refer to them as *ti doktè*, or "little doctor," a term that can be either disparaging or affectionate. Because many are from other parts of Haiti, they do not have the extensive local contacts and social networks that long-term personnel might be able to draw on. In addition, residents are not allowed to have other employment, which limits their income. These factors leave them in a somewhat precarious state. While certainly not confronted with the grinding struggles for survival that Haiti's poorest citizens are faced with, the residents often described their time at the Justinien as being particularly arduous, in terms of living and working conditions, workload, and pressure to fulfill a range of debts and obligations, particularly to their families and extended kin networks.

Admiration and Obligation

Training is a central component of the residents' lives and work. In theory, residents at the Justinien are to be trained by the hospital's attending physicians, who are supposed to conduct and participate in rounds, hold formal trainings and workshops for the residents, and supervise the latter's daily tasks and activities. In practice, however, the high rate of absenteeism among attending physicians meant that residents were left without any training or supervision. Notable exceptions included pediatrics and internal medicine, where physicians paid by Konbit Sante were explicitly responsible for training residents, and family medicine, a service that was created by faculty at an American university as a training program for residents in this branch of medicine. In other services, training was haphazard. Residents might benefit from the dedication and commitment to training by one or two physicians in the service, but for the most part were left to learn from textbooks, more senior residents, and their own experiences. While these residents had grown accustomed to the lack of supervision and mentorship from attending physicians, it remained a source of frustration and disappointment. Residents also resented that attending physicians received higher salaries with fewer delays in payment, despite the fact that residents' presence in and contributions to most services was much greater. One resident related an incident in which she approached a man in a ward and asked him rather aggressively why he was leafing through a patient's chart. His response, that he was an attending physician, embarrassed both of them—the resident, for having spoken to an attending physician in an abrupt manner, and the attending physician, for being unfamiliar to the resident despite the latter's constant presence in the service for over a year.

It is perhaps because of these configurations that those physicians who were present as supervisors and mentors were especially appreciated, and also why many residents told me that there were no physicians at the hospital whom they looked up to or who served as a model for their own professional aspirations. Others said that they had had a professor during medical school they admired, but that there were no models for them at the HUJ. Several told me that they would like to have the individual qualities of several physicians, but that there was no single doctor that they particularly admired. Those who did name a physician almost always named one from their own service, and certain physicians were named repeatedly by the residents. When I asked about admirable qualities that either characterized specific physicians or were appealing as abstract qualities, the residents gave a diversity of answers. Not surprisingly, residents appreciated those physicians who actively participated in their training and who acted as mentors. Residents explained that senior physicians who "take the time to explain things" and "don't keep what they know for themselves" were particularly appreciated. Other commonly mentioned qualities included attention and commitment to patient care, keeping up with current medical research and techniques (several residents used the English expression "up to date"), and finally, being able to manage interpersonal relationships. This involved not only being able to avoid or work through potentially conflictual situations but also to stick up for one's own interests and not be taken advantage of or pushed around by colleagues or superiors.

In terms of mentors, supervisors, and senior colleagues, young Haitian physicians today work with a reduced pool of health professionals due to decades of emigration. It is not uncommon, particularly in smaller clinics and dispensaries, for physicians fresh out of a yearlong internship to be the sole biomedical provider in the establishment, or in the case of very rural areas, the entire community. The residents, all of whom had completed a year of social service in a rural setting, often had negative memories of these experiences. They recalled being overwhelmed by the health conditions they confronted, the lack of resources available to address them, and being personally challenged by shortages of water, electricity, and at times, food. Isolation from family and friends meant not having access to the support networks that can and do cushion these kinds of hardships. Not having the mentorship, support, or advice of more senior physicians left them feeling incapacitated and discouraged, sentiments that I commonly heard expressed at the Justinien, despite its position as one of the country's largest health establishments and one of the few university teaching hospitals in Haiti. Meanwhile, colleagues who had emigrated, either before or during medical school, write back with reports of high salaries, access to sophisticated biomedical technologies and cutting-edge training, and a plethora of opportunities for intellectual growth and personal advancement.

Faced with mounting economic pressures, frustrated with their working conditions, and discouraged by the lack of mentorship and supervision, the residents decided to organize a strike to protest what they perceived to be the Haitian state's unwillingness to take their plight seriously.

The Residents on Strike

Compared to the standard of living of the majority of Haitians, the residents at the Justinien led a fairly comfortable existence. Approximately thirty had rooms on the second floor of a large building on the hospital's campus. Although the residents' rooms were fairly small, they had been recently refurbished after a fire had gutted the building in 2003. Each room had a single bed, a tile floor, and high ceilings. Communal bathrooms gave the residence the feeling of a college dormitory, and residents occasionally socialized in the rooms of their friends, although most of the time doors were shut, with residents either sleeping or working on the wards. Three small areas at the angle and each extremity of the L-shaped building were used for drying clothes, eating meals, and socializing.

This relatively comfortable appearance belied some major concerns that made residency at the Justinien a period of stress for young physicians. Foremost among these concerns were their salaries. The Ministry of Health allotted a stipend of approximately 200 USD per month per resident, a sum nearly seven times as much as the average per capita income in Haiti. With rapidly increasing costs of food, fuel, and daily goods, as well as rapid inflation (the residents were paid in Haitian gourdes) this amount was described as unreasonably low by all the residents, particularly in light of their level of education. For those with children and relatives to support, and those who had accumulated debt during their studies, economic pressures were a source of constant stress. In addition, stipend payments were often late, and residents regularly went for over six months without being paid. While they remained confident that the payments would arrive (and as I observed, they eventually did), working for months without income was chief among the residents' complaints.

The residents were also dissatisfied with their housing. While the building I just mentioned housed thirty residents, and some found lodging with relatives in the city, the remainder were housed in two other buildings—one that was equivalent to the main residence in terms of comfort and amenities, and the other which was much inferior. The *Kay Rat* (Rat House), as it was called, was above the patient wings in internal medicine. With its rotting wood floors and particle-board partition walls, it was indeed a haven for rats and other vermin. In addition, the residents' rooms were directly under the building's corrugated tin roof, which made their quarters unbearably hot for much of the year. All the residences were affected by frequent water and electricity shortages, and this was also a source of aggravation for the young physicians. Fetching water, whether for bathing, cooking, or drinking, is considered a particularly low-status task in Haiti, and is generally assigned to children or domestic servants, especially women. Since nearly all the residents lived away from their families and domestic workers, they would pay hospital employees to carry their water for them, or because of financial constraints, haul it themselves, a point of particular contention among the male residents. Electricity was used to power laptop computers, fans for ventilation, radios, and, in rare cases, televisions. While power outages were considered to be inconvenient and aggravating, all the residents seemed accustomed to them from before their arrival at the hospital, and they did not create as much anger and frustration as the water shortages.

Meals were also a key concern for the medical residents. While none of the young physicians suffered from food scarcity or insecurity in ways that resembled that of their poorer compatriots, access to regular, nutritious meals remained a challenge. Two couples of married residents lived in the residence with their children. Each couple had come to the hospital with two domestic workers who cooked in addition to doing laundry and providing childcare. A few other residents arranged with their colleagues (the domestic workers' employers) to have portions of food prepared for them as well. Others ate at nearby restaurants or food stands, while most made arrangements through a local caterer who had daily meals delivered. The caterer was understanding enough to accept deferred payment for meals, given the long wait for their stipends to come.

Living on credit was a particularly stressful and humiliating experience for the medical residents. By the time they had begun their residencies, they had already completed five years of medical school, one year of hospital-based internship, and a year of mandatory "service social," which generally involves work as a primary care physician in a public dispensary, clinic, or hospital. For the most part, they were in their mid to late twenties when they began their residencies and, to their families—who had supported their medical education and accompanied them during the challenging years of their training—they were already doctors. There was, henceforth, the expectation that the residents would transition from being *consumers of* to *contributors to* a family's resources, helping to pay for younger siblings' education, parents' housing and medical expenses, and other necessities.

In addition to their living conditions, the residents also found their working conditions to be unacceptable. As noted in previous chapters, despite being a large research hospital, the Justinien was plagued by deficient infrastructure and lacking in basic medical resources: electricity and running water were intermittent or absent on the wards; basic supplies such as bandages, medical instruments, and medications were insufficient; and basic procedures such as X-ray examinations or laboratory analyses were often unavailable. The residents were also critical of the labor practices and management at the hospital. In particular, they decried high rates of absenteeism among attending physicians and nurses with higher status, and a lack of oversight or authority in regard to job performance by the hospital's staff at large.

After months of not being paid, ongoing water shortages in the residences, and what they described as intolerable working conditions, the residents decided to go on strike. This decision was reached after a series of meetings in the residents' dining area. The extensive discussions were attended by nearly all the residents, and characterized by heated debates and occasional shouting, as well as outbursts of laughter. Charismatic residents, particularly those who were gifted in speaking and organizing rhetorical points, emerged as de facto spokespeople, while others took a more passive role in the negotiations, or simply stopped attending the meetings.

The strike was a moment when the residents' claims for better working conditions and what they considered to be a minimum standard of living for health care professionals were articulated through physical protest and impassioned discourse. To launch the strike, the residents held a press conference at the hospital. In addition to reading a statement that highlighted the factors motivating their actions, they also projected photographs intended to garner the journalists' sympathy. These included images of a male resident carrying water up the stairs to his dormitory, the decrepit and filthy bathrooms of the residents' lodging, and a resident performing a procedure on a patient at night by the light of a colleague's cell phone. It is not surprising that the journalists did indeed seem sympathetic to the young physicians' claims, given that the residents' complaints dovetailed with those of the general population in the identification both of the primary problem and its cause: a lack of resources that stemmed from an absent or dysfunctional state and the country's irresponsible and corrupt leaders.

At the beginning of the strike, the residents used a dramatic strategy to disrupt activities in the hospital's administrative offices. Approximately twenty of them entered the administration's reception area and, pounding buckets with sticks, beating the wooden benches with their hands, and scraping empty cans of infant formula on the cement floor, made such a deafening din that it was impossible to concentrate, much less accomplish any work or hold meetings. Some of the lower-level administrative staff who sympathized with the residents seemed to enjoy the rhythmic protest. One of the residents danced in a ring of noisemaking protesters. In their demonstration, the residents drew on several dimensions of Haitian performative protest, including call-and-response chanting (McAlister 2002). A leader yelled, "Bourik la . . ." (The donkey . . .) to which the others responded, "bouke!" (is exhausted!). The image of the donkey, the archetypical work animal in Haiti, was often used by the residents to describe their plight. Another chant involved a particularly unpopular administrator, who had expressed a callous insensitivity to the residents' requests for water by telling them that the ocean was just down the street. They nicknamed this administrator "Mànken" or "Model" because of his stylish and expensive wardrobe, and the chant described his incapacity and unwillingness to resolve basic problems. Even residents who were normally reserved and quiet enthusiastically joined in the chanting and pounded noisily on pots and furniture.[5]

The hospital administration's reaction to the strike was somewhat ambivalent but mostly supportive of the residents. While they did not take any actions that explicitly supported the strike, the Justinien's directors told me that it was understandable that such actions took place, given the long delays in receiving paychecks. However, they were unable to openly support the strike as doing so would have compromised their loyalty to their superiors at the Ministry of Health. Many of the hospital's regular physicians also supported the residents in their actions, but some were put off by the residents' use of a common Haitian proverb: "Bourik travay, chwal galonnen" (The donkey works, the horse gets the honors). Certain attending physicians did not appreciate this tacit critique of their absenteeism, and asked the residents to refrain from using this proverb in their protest. Nevertheless, the image of the donkey persisted in protest chants as well as on posters the residents made to hold up during demonstrations.

The strike lasted for just over a month. During this period, the residents employed a variety of protest tactics, including sitting on benches in front of the administrative offices (so that none of the staff could enter the building), standing and sitting in protest in front of the hospital gates so that no vehicles could enter the hospital grounds (during the seated protests, some of the residents played the board game Monopoly), and continuing to provide radio interviews to local and national journalists. Residents frequently mentioned that it was important to gain the local population's sympathy. Families of patients unable to access care at the hospital would be particularly opposed to the strike and possibly aggressive toward the residents, but the latter hoped that their claims for remuneration and decent working conditions would earn empathy and support. They crafted signs and placards that read: "Even if it looks like I'm well-dressed, I'm living on credit," "A stethoscope and a white coat aren't worth anything in the market," and "Klowòks is hard for everybody."[6]

The residents continued to meet to discuss their strategies throughout the strike, and many of their discussions centered on cases in which they should make exceptions and provide care. While all the residents agreed that care should not be withheld in cases where patients' lives were at risk, defining this criterion proved to be far from straightforward, and residents had differing interpretations of what they considered to be life-threatening conditions. Some residents were not supportive of the strike at all, feeling that their professional status obligated them to provide care despite the delays in remuneration. Others were concerned that the interruption in their work would lead to an extension of their residency and delay its completion. (This proved to be a valid concern, when many of the

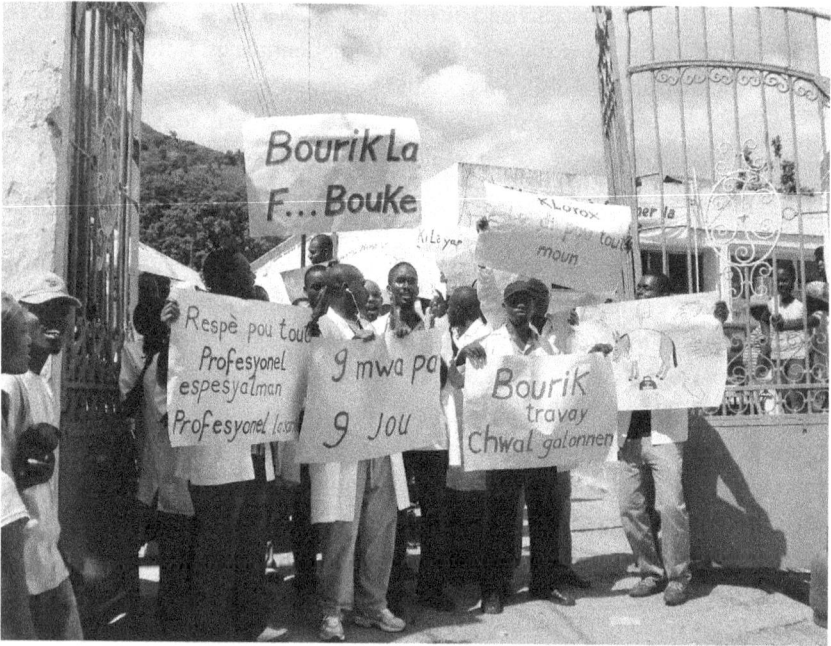

FIGURE 3.1.   Medical residents protest at the gates of the Hôpital Universitaire Justinien. Their signs (starting at the top and moving clockwise) read: "The donkey is f . . . ing exhausted," "*Klorox* is hard for everyone," "The donkey works, the horse is decorated," "9 months aren't 9 days," "Respect for all professionals, especially health professionals." The sign at the far right shows a donkey in a white coat with a stethoscope around its neck, and a medical bag on the ground, being pointed at by accusatory fingers. October 2008. Photo by the author.

department heads did in fact extend the length of residencies to compensate for the work time that was lost during the strike.) For the most part, however, the residents were united in their strike for the five weeks of its duration. It ended when the Ministry of Health sent checks to residents that covered six out of ten months of back pay. During the strike, medical activities at the hospital decreased significantly. Nurses complained to me that they had to work longer hours to compensate for the residents' absence, but I did not notice any increase in the presence of attending physicians during the strike.

The strike led to a major disruption in the hospital's services and to the very visible and public expression of residents' frustration, dissatisfaction, and claims on the hospital's administration and the Haitian state. Rather than responding to an exception or unusual situation, however, the residents reacted to a series of chronic deficiencies and challenges that characterized their work before and after the strike, and that are widespread in public health establishments throughout

Haiti. In the years following the 2008 strike, work stoppages have become wide-spread in public hospitals and health centers in Haiti. In 2016 a nationwide strike of health workers in the public health system lasted nearly five months, causing a major reduction in services available to the population (Honoré et al. 2016). While these strikes were not directed at international agencies or organizations, they occur in public establishments that often have partnerships with such groups, and whose activities are affected by the work stoppages.

While the residents at the Justinien were much more likely to fault Haiti's Ministry of Health and the Haitian government more broadly than international entities for their plight, they nonetheless had had extensive and critical reflections on the place of foreign interventions in Haiti's biomedical health services.

Reflections on Foreign Aid

When I asked the residents about their involvement with international aid, they initially minimized their contacts and relationships. Oftentimes, they situated themselves as mere observers or witnesses: "I see them come through the hospital and drop things off, but I've never talked with them or asked where they're from." One whose residency program was designed, funded, and implemented by a foreign group told me, "We're not really involved with them, sometimes when they give trainings . . . what else? . . . I do what they ask us to do in the unit, we give care to people with HIV/AIDS, but direct ties, I can't say that we have any." Many began by insisting that they had no contact whatsoever with foreign aid in any form, but when I prompted them by naming specific groups or interventions, they acknowledged their presence and activities in their services. While not all residents encounter foreign aid workers on a daily basis (although many do), all are involved in international interventions of some form in their work. Involvement may include prescribing or dispensing donated medications and goods, using donated equipment, working in facilities built with foreign funds, implementing programs designed by international agencies, working alongside foreign medical staff, or attending foreign-sponsored or foreign-led trainings both in Haiti and abroad.

There are two factors that I believe explain why Haitian health care workers minimize their contact with international interventions. The first is that many of these interventions are so pervasive throughout medical establishments in Haiti that they are not considered noteworthy. All the vaccines that I saw at the hospital, for example, had been donated by international agencies and governments, yet were never named by informants as a form of foreign intervention. Donated medications and equipment, buildings sponsored by foreign funds, paperwork and forms designed and printed by international agencies and NGOs, these all formed a part of the residents' daily work environment, and while they would recognize them as international in origin if I asked about them specifically, they rarely named them when asked in more general terms. This even applied to foreign aid workers. After a resident would tell me that they had no contact with any form of international medical aid, I would ask if they had any Cubans working in their service, to which they would often respond by exclaiming, "Oh, yes, we do! I forgot about the Cubans!"

The second factor that may explain Haitian health care workers' tendency to minimize or downplay the presence of international interventions in their places of work has to do with a more widespread phenomenon I observed among people in Haiti: that of being discrete about and in some cases disparaging of available resources. As I have discussed in previous chapters, there are pragmatic and discursive reasons that make it advantageous for the recipients of aid to deny the existence or minimize the importance of existing sources of support, specifically because doing so may increase the chances of obtaining additional resources. The totalizing pronouncements that I described as rhetorical negation were common in the residents' discourses: "This isn't a hospital! A hospital wouldn't run like this, it wouldn't be in this condition!"; "We don't have a government in Haiti, we don't have leaders"; "There's nothing good left in Haiti." Claiming that there were no international interventions or support in their respective departments would strengthen the residents' commonly repeated claim that the Justinien had no redeeming qualities.

While nearly all the residents initially minimized their own contact with international medical aid, all acknowledged that such aid was present in the hospital, and when asked to elaborate, almost all of them began by describing the work of Konbit Sante (with the exception of the residents in the family medicine training program sponsored by the Florida-based university, who spoke first of that program). As mentioned in the previous chapter, descriptions of Konbit Sante and its activities often focused on the group's provision of materials and supplies. Other foreign interventions that were commonly named included those that involved a variety of the hospital's departments, such as the US government's PEPFAR program and its provision of HIV treatments and services, or the visiting teams of American and Dominican orthopedists whose weeklong stays in the hospital's main operating room affected all of the hospital's surgical activities. Finally, many residents mentioned programs that involved opportunities for them to travel abroad for training: Konbit Sante has facilitated travel to Maine for several members of the hospital's staff and administration, including medical residents, and a small number of French universities have offered internship opportunities for anesthesiology and internal medicine residents. As these interventions were not only specifically directed at residents but also represented extremely desirable opportunities for them, it is not surprising that they were mentioned by many of my informants. Other initiatives, such as smaller projects that targeted a single service, were rarely mentioned.

In addition to contact with international interventions through their work at the hospital, nearly all the residents had spent some time abroad, not only for training or student exchanges but also to visit relatives and friends, mostly in North America. During my research, two residents traveled to the United States in the later stages of their pregnancies, giving birth to babies who qualified for US citizenship and strengthening the transnational ties that offered the promise of future emigration. Residents had also had contact with international partnerships during medical school (approximately one-third of them had participated in a month-long rotation at a French medical school in Guadeloupe); during their year of social service in health establishments (mostly in public hospitals and clinics, but these often had international interventions present in them); or during residency itself, when residents in family practice, pediatrics, and surgery had monthlong rotations in various NGO-run hospitals throughout the country. Their reflections on these latter experiences are particularly telling.

I asked the residents to compare their experiences working in health establishments operated by international NGOs and the Justinien. All who were in a position to make this comparison agreed that the work environments were very different. They focused on two main points. The first was that, in foreign-run, private hospitals, materials and resources were available when needed, both in terms of specialized equipment and medicines and in terms of basic resources for patients. Residents remarked that patients received care and basic services even if they did not have the means to pay, whereas this was not the case in public establishments. The second point was related to management. Most of my informants who had worked in NGO-run hospitals claimed that the management was better than in the public system. As one resident told me, "In the state system, you often get the impression that the medical staff often do whatever they want. But in NGO hospitals, one has to do exactly what they ask of you, from the intake to discharge." While some emphasized that NGO-run hospitals have their own problems and shortcomings (one resident told me that she had not been particularly impressed by any of the four NGO hospitals she had worked at), the consensus was that health care facilities operated by foreign NGOs offered better services for patients and better working conditions for staff than public facilities did. Despite this relatively positive assessment, the residents offered an ambivalent analysis when asked to describe the motivations of foreigners carrying out medical interventions in Haiti.

Reading Motivations

When I asked the residents what they thought motivated foreigners to come to carry out medical interventions in Haiti, most respondents began by stating that they were unsure. A few, particularly those with whom I had less rapport or were less comfortable with being interviewed, refused to even conjecture, simply saying that they did not and could not know. The majority, however, continued by telling me they thought that there were two types of people who came to Haiti to do medical work. The first were described in terms such as "people who really want to help us"; "those who see how many problems we have and are motivated by the suffering they see"; "people who come in with good will and want things to change." These motivations were described in matter-of-fact terms. The residents did not elaborate on their responses, speculate on the origins of these motivations, or associate them with a specific nationality or religion.

The second group described by the residents consisted of people who came to Haiti for other reasons. Foremost among these was personal financial gain. Salaries paid to Haitians by international bodies, particularly NGOs, tend to be significantly higher than those paid by the government of Haiti. Specifically in the health field, work with international employers is considered to be particularly lucrative; it is not surprising, therefore, that the residents associated work with international agencies with lucrative pay. In addition, international aid workers often have access to luxuries such as private vehicles and expensive hotels, none of which are within the reach of the majority of people in Haiti, not even for many health care workers who earn relatively higher incomes. As one resident told me, "Ils viennent pour faire leur beurre" (They come to make their butter). None of the residents I spoke with claimed that foreign aid workers' activities in Haiti should *not* be remunerated—their objections centered more on the discrepancy between claims of assisting others while acting principally out of self-interest. There were also some who observed that foreigners' salaries were disproportionately high when compared with the wages earned by Haitian health professionals.

Another motivation cited by several residents was foreigners' desire to see exotic or unusual pathologies. Those who spoke of this issue generally told me of a firsthand encounter working with a foreigner or group of foreigners who became visibly excited when seeing cases of infectious diseases such as malaria or dengue. In the words of one resident: "There are some who are happy to see cases that they don't see in their own country. I was at a hospital where we were examining a patient who had an intestinal perforation caused by typhus. The foreigner next to me said, 'Wow! It's like in the books!'" Many of the international medical aid volunteers and workers who travel to Haiti usually work in relatively affluent communities, where infectious diseases and other ailments linked to extreme poverty may be relatively rare, or where pathologies and injuries will be treated at an earlier state, rather than developing into more serious and extreme conditions as they often do in Haiti. In addition, many are either older professionals who seldom confront unfamiliar pathologies in their own practices, or younger students and clinicians who are particularly enthusiastic about opportunities to encounter a wide range of pathologies. As trainees themselves, the Haitian medical residents I interviewed could relate to the pedagogical potential offered by exotic pathologies.

Other motivations for foreigners to practice medicine in Haiti that were named by the residents included the possibility of trying out experimental therapies. One resident claimed: "They come to do experiments. Where they come from, there are so many regulations, there are things they can't do there." Foreigners were also thought to be sent to Haiti to help control infectious diseases that could threaten their own countries, or simply to be seen doing good works, with the implication that the visibility of the action was more important than its substance. In addition to suspecting that not all foreigners who came to Haiti to carry out medical interventions were motivated by altruism, a similar ambivalence applied to material donations. Residents frequently complained that broken, useless, and expired equipment and supplies were sent to Haiti because the sending country had no use for them, while others commented that donors could obtain tax rebates for doing so. Several suggested that it might be easier to send the refuse to Haiti rather than dispose of it domestically.

Even those residents who did not name specific unsavory motivations commented that they doubted that all foreign aid in Haiti was motivated by altruism, both in the case of medical aid, and in terms of international interventions more generally. The evidence supporting these doubts was clear and simple: worsening conditions throughout the country. As one resident explained: "It's as though they're not really helping, because the problems are still there. We have plenty of organizations that are 'helping' in this or that area, but we get the impression that the organizations make it so that the problems stay, so that they can stay and profit." In addition to the sheer number of international organizations and agencies active throughout Haiti, residents often mentioned that they were constantly hearing news reports about large sums of money that had been pledged or delivered by international bodies. Why, they wondered, are conditions getting worse if so many resources are purportedly directed toward improving them? These worsening conditions, even before the catastrophic events of 2010, were prime factors in motivating their intent to go, as Dr. Célestin put it, "where they need me."

Emigration and the "Brain Drain"

Emigration is a constant theme in the lives of Haitian professionals. While a desire to travel abroad is commonly expressed by young Haitians of all socioeconomic classes, young professionals usually have many relatives and colleagues who have already migrated, and most seem to be actively exploring avenues for migration. Out of the fifty-two residents I interviewed, only two told me that they did not intend to leave Haiti to pursue careers abroad. The majority told me that they planned to go to the United States (although several named Canada and France as desirable destinations) and many were preparing to take the United States Medical Licensing Examination (USMLE) that would permit them to qualify for an American residency program. Based on the experiences of family members and colleagues, many anticipated that emigration could involve a decline in their professional status. Some planned to work in nursing or other health-related professions, and a few planned to leave the medical domain entirely. The residents often heard and repeated anecdotes of doctors, nurses, lawyers, and teachers who left Haiti and, due to factors ranging from racism and xenophobia to the challenges of learning a foreign language and adapting to a new society, became taxi drivers, maids, and manual laborers in North America. Despite these risks, the residents were encouraged by stories of migrants' spectacular successes and disheartened by the prospects of remaining in a country that "pa ofri nou anyen" (doesn't offer us anything).

The term *brain drain* was first used in the 1960s by scholars examining the movement of educated and skilled professionals from Western Europe to the United States (Grubel and Scott 1977, 3–4). For many years, it was used in straightforward terms: the departure of scientists, engineers, health professionals, and brilliant students represented a loss for the sending country, particularly impoverished nations lacking in skilled workers and basic infrastructure. In recent years, however, the concept has been critiqued, and new terms have been introduced to add nuance to analyses of migration. The expression *brain gain* was coined to describe the benefits for sending countries that often accompany the emigration of skilled professionals, including remittances, return migration, and diaspora networks.[7] *Brain circulation* highlights the continual movement of migration professionals, who, rather than migrating a single time from a poorer country to a wealthier one, are involved in lifelong movements and exchanges across national borders (R. Patterson 2007). *Brain waste* is used to describe the inability of professionals to reap the benefits commensurate with their education and talent, whether it is in their home country (due to lack of infrastructure or emigration possibilities) or abroad after migration (Mattoo, Neagu, and Özden 2005). Finally, scholars have developed expressions such as *the international mobility of talent* (Solimano 2008).

Most writing on brain drain and its related concepts is done by economists, policy analysts, and political scientists. Anjali Sahay (2009) divides this literature into the following categories: studies of the causes of professionals' migration; analyses that attempt to determine the scope and magnitude of this migration; and literature examining the impact and consequences of this migration on sending and receiving countries. He also points out that most of these studies are hypothetical, as reliable data on this issue is difficult to obtain (particularly from sending countries) and almost none of the studies obtain information from migrating professionals themselves (22).

While the writers who promote the concept of brain gain point to the advantages the emigration of professionals can have for countries of origin (particularly in the form of remittances and other economic contributions), they often mention the departure of health professionals as an example of its disadvantages. After describing cases where migrant entrepreneurs and venture capitalists built bridges for the transfer of technologies, information, and resources between wealthy nations and their countries of origin, Solimano (2008) continues:

> However, not all talent mobility is as glamorous as these examples suggest. A particularly dramatic case is the massive and persistent emigration of medical doctors, nurses, and other workers in the health sector coming from poor nations in Sub-Saharan Africa, from the Philippines and other developing countries who go to work to the UK, US, Canada, Australia, and other developed countries. The negative side effect of this mobility of health professionals is the weakening of the health sector in the source countries. This is particularly serious in the case of Africa, suffering from an AIDS epidemic, malaria, and other diseases that cause loss of human life and impair countries' development potential. This poses conflicts between the private interests of health professionals and the social needs of the health sector in the home countries. (3)

These conflicts are apparent in Haiti, where an absence of health care workers is decried by Haitian and international observers and commentators, while Haitian professionals emphasize the lack of opportunities and future prospects in their home country.

As Haitian medical residents plan their emigration and anticipated integration into a foreign health care system, they are inspired by memories of experiences abroad (only two of the fifty-two residents interviewed had never left Haiti). The others had traveled to North America, France, and other Caribbean islands, either to visit friends and relatives, or as part of training during medical school. Those who had spent time in hospitals abroad (primarily in France or the French territories of Guadeloupe and Martinique, as part of a university exchange) described the experience as very positive, despite some difficulties adapting to a foreign setting and negative encounters with racist colleagues. They were impressed by the level of technological sophistication they encountered in foreign hospitals, as well as the functioning of the establishments they worked in. In the words of a surgery resident: "There were a lot of things that I was seeing for the first time. It was my first experience with scanners, and learning how to read them. Their medical system also really appealed to me, how well everything was managed and controlled." A resident who had spent two months in Montreal during medical school said, "I like the Canadian health care system so much that I want to go back to it. It helps clinicians who want to learn more, and the academic support is really amazing."

In addition to exposing them to promising work environments, these experiences also increased residents' frustrations and dismay when they returned to Haiti and realized how little, in comparative terms, was available in terms of diagnostic equipment, range of treatments, and resources for patient care. One resident told me,

> I did a six-week training in Guadeloupe, and it let me see how far we have to go in Haiti. I was at a little clinic, but they have everything, *everything*, it's well-organized, it's terrific. We [in Haiti] are really far from the way that medicine should be practiced. What we do here has some value, because we save lives. It's as though we're doing war medicine. We're always in an emergency. Guadeloupe is small, but they're well-organized. Why aren't we? Is it an issue of bad faith, I don't know. But it angered me to see everything that they're doing in Guadeloupe, so close to us, while we're just treading water.

For some of the residents, their experiences in hospitals abroad allowed for first-hand encounters with the practice of medical specialties that are not available in Haiti, areas such as laparoscopic surgery or neurology. In these cases, emigration was associated with the possibility of training and practice in these domains.

The residents' primary reason for wishing to leave Haiti was to pursue economic opportunities abroad. While many also mentioned the desire to further their education and concerns related to insecurity in Haiti, it is ultimately the hope of higher salaries and improved standards of living that attract young Haitian physicians to the United States, Canada, France, and elsewhere. It should be noted, however, that Haitian migrants' salaries are often used to support family in Haiti—remittances from overseas migrants, (estimated at over 3 billion USD annually) constitute a significant portion of Haiti's revenue, surpassing formal aid and income from exports (US Department of State 2010).[8] When these young physicians migrate, it is very likely that they will support their kin network as they themselves have been supported by relatives abroad. Several residents told me explicitly that the higher salaries they would earn abroad would contribute to household income in Haiti, and could be directed toward expenses such as school fees for younger siblings or cousins or medical care for aging parents. The prevalence of remittances in Haitian household economies contribute to residents' convictions that they could contribute more to their home country by emigrating than by remaining there. Nina Glick Schiller and Georges Fouron (2001), who examined Haitian Americans' sense of obligation toward relatives and kin in Haiti, write about a "morality of knowledge," through which migrants' firsthand knowledge of conditions in the country they have left behind serves as grounds for efforts to help remedy the situation. They claim that, in the context of migration and obligation, "a person's humanity is defined by their acts of helping others" (66). As one of their informants explained, "Naturally, it's an obligation [to support people in Haiti]. It is because you left your close relatives here in poverty. The people you left behind must survive, and you must have a certain humanity in your heart. You are obligated to send a little something for that person to survive. . . . That is a necessity because you left them and you know what conditions they are living in" (78).

Many residents spoke of migration as a temporary strategy that would lead to an eventual return to Haiti. The resident who had traveled to Montreal told me,

> These days, I'm really disgusted by the system here, and that gives me momentum to go back [to Canada], to take the equivalency exams. But that momentum hasn't killed my desire to work for my country. I need to go get some experience, to be sure. I need to make enough money, come back here, and set up a serious hospital, one that complies with international regulations, so that patients don't have to be responsible for getting sheets for their beds or getting food to eat. But for now, after my residency in Haiti, I think I'll spend at most a year or two in Haiti, then I'll leave to get some experience abroad, and after a while, come back to my country to settle down.

Such narratives are common among Haitian migrants, whose departure from Haiti does not preclude continued involvement in the country's economic, political, and social life, either as residents abroad, or as eventual returnees to Haiti (Glick Schiller and Fouron 2001). In most cases, migrants choose whether or not they will remain involved in affairs in Haiti, and what form this involvement might take. In some cases, however, this involvement is determined by a contractual agreement.

International Aid and Contractual Return

In addition to working with resources donated by international agencies and working alongside foreign clinicians in their workplaces, young Haitian health workers encounter international aid in a form that has the possibility of transforming their careers and lives: training programs sponsored by foreign governments and organizations. With the training of health professionals in impoverished settings identified as a priority by a growing number of international actors, more foreign organizations and governments are providing training for Haitian health professionals, both in the country and abroad. These programs are intended to remedy a dearth of opportunities for aspiring health workers in the Haitian education system. Entrance into Haiti's medical and nursing schools is extremely competitive, with very few openings compared to the number of applicants. Once students have completed high school (which already represents a significant expense for most Haitian families), they face a number of obstacles if they hope to obtain post-secondary education. Not only must university students pay significant tuition fees (with the exception of the state university, whose fees are nominal) but those who come from outside Port-au-Prince must also relocate and find housing in the capital. (All of Haiti's four accredited medical schools are located in Port-au-Prince, as are many of its nursing schools.) Students also struggle to cover expenses associated with their studies: transportation, textbooks, photocopied texts, laptop computers and maintenance, and associated items such as hospital scrubs and a stethoscope. Once these expenses are covered, university students face other challenges. I often heard criticism about the quality of medical education from Haitians trained in the system as well as from international observers. Major problems include a lack of pedagogical resources, professor absenteeism, interruptions due to strikes and instability, and a focus on theoretical training that leaves students without sufficient practical experience. For all of these reasons, international bodies, both governmental and nongovernmental, have been active in training Haitian health care workers through a variety of initiatives.

The best-known and largest of these programs (in terms of number of students) is sponsored by Cuba. In 2004 the Cuban government, as part of its ongoing effort to support Haiti's Ministry of Health and its establishments, began offering free medical education to select Haitian high school graduates. The program aims to recruit students from throughout the country, and chooses candidates through a competitive examination held in all ten of Haiti's departments. Approximately one hundred students are chosen annually based on examination scores (as well as a much smaller number based on the discretion of officials in Haiti's Ministry of Health); they receive five years of medical education, housing, and board at the Escuela Latinoamericana de Medicina's campus in Santiago de Cuba. There, they form one of the largest groups of international students among a cohort that includes students from Africa, Latin America, and a small number from North America. As part of this arrangement, Haitian students must sign a contract that obligates them to return to practice medicine in a public establishment in their area of origin for at least five years.

Other, smaller-scale training initiatives include scholarships from churches or private organizations that will sponsor a promising student's medical training in Haiti, programs through foreign universities that will host a Haitian student for periods ranging from two weeks to several years, and programs in Haiti such as the Justinien's family medicine resident training program, which offers advanced medical training for students in Haiti by drawing on the resources of a foreign institution or government (in this case, an American university, USAID, and other funders). These programs may or may not have a contractual clause included in their arrangements that secures the trainees' staying in or returning to Haiti upon completing the training. Enforcing these agreements is not always simple—I was told of one case where a private American foundation paid for a medical student's medical education in Haiti in exchange for the student's commitment to work at the foundation's rural hospital. The foundation pressed criminal charges when the graduate refused to fulfill his contractual obligations. Eventually, the case was resolved when the young physician reimbursed the foundation for the cost of his studies.

I asked the medical residents for their perspectives on subsidized medical training in exchange for a commitment to work in Haiti. None of the residents had signed a contractual agreement to remain in Haiti after their training, but two of the largest groups of residents, those in family medicine and those in pediatrics, were in programs that were funded by foreign organizations (a university in Florida and Konbit Sante) whose support of the residency was explicitly intended to contribute to the Haitian medical workforce. In the case of the family medicine program, the residency was designed with the explicit aim of encouraging trainees to work in rural and underserved settings. The residents were aware of this dimension of the program, but their opinions on these issues remained personal and pragmatic. More than abstract reflections on debt and obligation, the thoughts they shared with me focused primarily on pragmatic concerns:

> RESIDENT: Unfortunately, a doctor has needs to live too, he can't just sit anywhere. That's why most family doctors work for NGOs. . . . They have scanners, they have equipment. And that's where they really play the role of family doctors, they see people, and after, they call on

specialists. The state should organize things this way. But family doctors are all in NGOs or private practice, the state doesn't use them. The state hasn't hired a single one of us yet.

PM: Would a doctor accept to go work in a rural area if there's a good salary, even if there might not be infrastructure, or good schools in the area?

RESIDENT: If there's enough money, he'll work something out. He can see his family on weekends. Because his heart was formed for work. That's what we're trained for, for rural work.

The residents made explicit ties between living conditions for medical professionals and state responsibility. A resident explained to me:

> The state has to make conditions suitable for them to stay. They're not leaving because they don't love their country, because they don't love their brothers, but because the conditions aren't there. Your whole family has its eyes on you. You're an investment for it, your little brothers and sisters. The conditions have to be there for you to be able to work and look after people's needs. If the conditions aren't there, if there's no water, no electricity, they don't pay you well. . . . I think those are the reasons why doctors leave. If it weren't like that, doctors would stay in their communities and give service, they would stay, and help others. Abroad, it's good, people respect your work. But it's not without sacrifice, because sometimes you feel like they humiliate you, you feel like you're not at home. You're more appreciated in your own country, by the patients. The leaders don't appreciate you at all, they don't respect you, they don't understand that if you work you need to eat, drink, to have electricity and water. I think those conditions exist abroad, but not here. It's not because they don't love their country. It's because the state doesn't take its responsibilities. What you don't find here you'll find elsewhere.

While most of the residents were opposed to the establishment of contractual agreements stipulating a trainee's return to Haiti, a few supported the practice while dismissing its relevance for their own lives:

> RESIDENT: Those programs are good, because usually, given the little that's offered here, we lose the benefits [of training health care workers], we always have the same problem. Foreign countries have enough, here, we're lacking. It's a good thing, something to promote. Haitian doctors have to be encouraged to stay in the country, and we'll have improvements in health.

PM: Would you have signed this kind of agreement?

RESIDENT: I already have a desire to stay, whether or not there's a contract. A contract isn't what's going to make me stay, I *know* that I have to stay.

While this resident was one of the two I interviewed who hoped to stay in Haiti and work for an NGO, she confided that her husband, also a physician, was preparing to take the USMLE.

Other concerns expressed by the residents included what they perceived as limited opportunities for intellectual and academic growth if they were to stay in Haiti. In the words of a pediatrics resident: "To tell us that we have to stay here after only getting this training? No way. We have to go see how things are better elsewhere, we have things to learn." This concern was also reflected in comments about what many residents perceived to be "real medicine."

Real Medicine

A recurring theme among Haitian medical residents was the difference between the medicine they practiced on a daily basis at the Justinien as compared to the medical practices they had experienced during periods abroad, or to a lesser extent, in private establishments in Haiti. During trips to Paris, Miami, or Montreal, they had seen "la vraie médecine" (real medicine) or "la médecine du 21ième siècle" (twenty-first-century medicine). In contrast, as one resident told me, "We're doing twentieth-century medicine. I don't even know if I could call it that. This isn't medicine at all." For most of the residents, the primary difference involved access to sophisticated biomedical technological equipment and the availability of medical materials in general. Coming from a hospital where the single X-ray machine was inoperative for months at a time, working in an environment with complex monitors, sophisticated scanners, and a seemingly endless variety of laboratory exams made a strong impression on the young Haitian doctors. While Haitian physicians are recognized by their Western colleagues for being outstanding at empirical diagnosis due to the lack of laboratory tests and equipment, they also experience the frustration of not being certain that they have made a correct diagnosis. "We have to start treatment and hope it works," one physician told me, "but often the patient doesn't return and we never know what she had." Overall, the residents' descriptions of the "real medicine" they encountered abroad focused on the presence and availability of sophisticated biomedical technologies, and their use to diagnose or treat conditions that may have been impossible to address in Haiti. "It's like what we learn about in our studies, but never get to do in practice," one resident told me. In addition, they were struck by the availability of more basic supplies and equipment that allowed them to do their work. Working in a foreign operating room and having the appropriate surgical equipment on hand meant not having to fish around in a bin and find an approximation of the desired tool as they regularly had to do at the Justinien. Even in sites that were considered underresourced or where patients lacked medical insurance, basic medical supplies such as antiseptics, gauze, and medications for primary care seemed unlimited, unlike in Haiti.

An ironic dimension of the residents' formulations of medicine abroad as "real medicine" is that they were mirrored by many of the medical aid volunteers who come to Haiti from wealthier countries. I often heard these volunteers describe their activities in Haiti as being more valuable and worthwhile than their medical activities in their home countries. Encountering and treating dramatic or life-threatening conditions such as neglected congenital deformations, lethal diseases, and severely debilitating pathologies were described by these informants as "real medicine" in comparison to the routine, chronic, and relatively benign pathologies many of them encountered in their home practices. Such discourse related to authenticity and impact frequently appears in the promotional materials of aid groups and organizations, which encourage potential aid volunteers, workers, and supporters to "change a life," "save a child," and "make a real difference." While foreign health professionals in Haiti are often perturbed by the lack of resources and technology available there, I have also heard several state that working in such conditions allows for the emergence and development of "real" medical skills, such as diagnosis based on direct observation and treatments that rely on practitioners' resourcefulness and flexibility. Working in difficult conditions was also described by some foreign clinicians as a test of one's commitment to medical practice and the well-being of patients, particularly if the latter were not able to remunerate the person caring for them.

"We're Waiting for the Foreigners!"

Focusing our attention on young Haitian physicians' interactions with and perspectives on international health interventions can reveal much about humanitarian and global health projects that are not apparent at first glance. Two encounters between Haitian physicians, their patients, and their foreign colleagues are particularly telling. In the first instance, a resident at the Justinien told me about an experience she had had while on a monthlong rotation at an American-run rural hospital, one that regularly receives groups of clinicians from the United States on weeklong medical missions. When the resident began calling out patients' names in the waiting room to begin her day of consultations, no one responded. After calling several names to no response, she asked the waiting crowd what was going on. "N ap tann blan yo!" (We're waiting for the foreigners!), someone called out. The resident laughed as she told me this anecdote, but it was clear that she had been wounded by the episode. While the majority of residents' complaints about feeling underappreciated involved the state, the country's leaders, and the hospital's administration, several residents complained about patients not "giving our work any value." This episode was particularly hurtful since the resident felt she had far more experience with the kinds of pathologies that typically brought patients to the rural hospital than did the foreign clinicians, and would be able to communicate more directly and effectively with them.

Foreign clinicians, particularly those who came to Haiti for short stays, were often not aware of these dynamics, as many of these comments and conversations happened discretely and in Creole. In the second instance, however, I witnessed an American team hearing from a translator that a patient refused to see the team's Haitian partner physician, but wanted to see a foreign doctor instead. After an uncomfortable silence, an American nurse indignantly told the translator: "Well, you tell her that if she doesn't want to see Dr. Jean-Louis, she can just go home!" The nurse recognized the slight toward her Haitian colleague and expressed indignation on his behalf.

While there are certainly instances in which Haitian patients would prefer to see a Haitian health care worker because of familiarity, trust, and ease of communication, the valorization of medicine from abroad as "real medicine" extends beyond Haitian physicians to the patients themselves. Medical care from abroad is viewed by many Haitians as being of higher quality and more effective, particularly if one has unsuccessfully sought care from local practitioners. While the desire to access resources that originate in a place of power and prestige is understandable, it is not without consequences. For example, a hospital administrator complained to me about the fact that patients would often delay seeking care (for periods of several months) in a Haitian clinic or hospital knowing that a foreign team would be coming to the area eventually. In addition to bemoaning the fact that such groups often did not keep reliable records and had little knowledge of local pathologies or treatments, she also criticized them for dispensing not only medical services for free but also food, clothing, and school supplies. The administrator felt that such practices led to unrealistic expectations of or resentment toward establishments such as the one she directed, which charged nominal consultation fees and attempted to limit the amount of material goods they dispensed to patients in an effort to decrease dependency.

The work of Haitian health professionals is shaped by emotions and reflections that are as diverse as the institutions they work with. Despite developing sophisticated critiques of international aid and the economic and geopolitical systems in which it operates, they are also aware that without the influx of resources, their work and professional aspirations would not be possible. Rather than having a single reaction vis-à-vis the foreign humanitarian projects that target their country, Haitian physicians' affective appraisals of aid are complex, ambivalent, and at times contradictory. Research in other settings suggests that many of the dynamics I have described here are not unique to Haiti. Alice Street (2014) found that Papuan doctors both resented and felt valorized by the exchanges they maintained with kin in their home villages, while simultaneously participating in transnational exchange networks of aid, training, and research that situated them on the margins of global medicine. Claire Wendland (2010) found that Malawian medical students had a similar idea that "real medicine was what happened elsewhere" (135). Rather than culturally bound reactions, research in this area suggests that humanitarian biomedical interventions and global health may be producing similar subjectivities and relations across diverse settings. In the next chapter, I examine how articulating the concept of moral economy may be useful for examining some of the less visible dimensions of medical aid, a process that allows for comparative perspectives between Haiti and other sites.

4

COMPONENTS OF A MORAL ECONOMY

In his article "Moral Economies Revisited," the anthropologist and physician Didier Fassin claims that the seminal concept of moral economy's "banalization tends to weaken its analytic acuity" (Fassin 2009, 1240). Later in the same text, he characterizes it as a "concept in becoming" and highlights its "analytic potential and critical strength" (2009, 1266, my translation). These seemingly paradoxical positions are indicative of the ambivalence many scholars feel toward moral economy, including E. P. Thompson himself, the British historian credited with first developing the concept in the 1960s (Thompson 1963; 1971; 1991, 271). On the one hand, moral economy offers a tool for investigating calculations, assessments, and transfers that lie outside the scope of conventional economics as well as an analytic framework for morality and ethics that assumes change and interaction rather than static codes or precepts. This appeal is tempered, on the other hand, by wariness of the term's vagueness and its propensity for engulfing all dimensions of human interaction, thereby rendering it, as Fassin fears, analytically dull. In this chapter, I suggest that one method for strengthening the concept's analytic potential and increasing its relevance for anthropology is to think of a moral economy in terms of its components. Using a straightforward definition of a moral economy, I consider how three of these components—interest, credit, and debt—can reveal some of the more subtle dimensions of transnational processes in Haiti's health care system.

Of Morality and Economics

Because Didier Fassin (2009) and Mark Edelman (2005) have provided detailed and insightful genealogies of a moral economy, I will not repeat this background here but simply identify the themes and debates that have characterized the concept's use. Since E. P. Thompson initially used it to describe the actions and reactions of the English populace to perceived injustice in the eighteenth century, a moral economy has been invoked and critiqued by historians, political scientists, sociologists, and anthropologists focusing on many periods and contexts. As Fassin notes, much of the concept's limitation stems from the fact that many contemporary authors present it as a given without clarifying its scope or constitution (Fassin 2009, 1256). Notable exceptions include studies of agrarian economic systems and processes of governance, where the legacies of Thompson's (1963, 1971, 1991) and James Scott's (1976) analyses are particularly influential. David Griffith uses North Carolina tobacco farmers' portrayal of their work as a "morally valuable enterprise" to argue that "moral-economic principles continue to be at work in advanced capitalist settings" (2009, 433). In a similar vein, Edelman (2005) argues for the continued relevance of Scott's moral economy analyses, specifically in relation to twenty-first-century transnational peasant movements in a globalized world. For these authors and others drawing from the same intellectual tradition, a moral economy is primarily a matter of sentiment and sensibility that involves the affective reactions of subaltern populations facing powerful adversaries who continue to occupy a central place in their analyses. Although this chapter builds on this literature, I aim to illustrate the relevance of a moral economy to spheres other than production and consumption and to populations—in this case, Haitian clinicians and expatriate aid workers—whose subaltern status is not without ambiguities.

While moral-economic principles are certainly evident in Haiti's embattled agricultural sector, a widespread scarcity of resources, the density of social relations, and an explicit preoccupation with morality and moral behaviors make other realms of daily life just as salient for these types of analyses. Erica James, drawing on fieldwork conducted in Port-au-Prince during the late 1990s, describes the intersecting "terror economies" and "compassion economies" that resulted from the 1991 to 1994 coup regime in Haiti and the transnational military and humanitarian interventions that followed. Terror economies were generated through "acts of intimidation, destruction of property, theft, torture, and murder" (2010, 26). In response, compassion economies consisted of "finite flows of beneficent material resources, knowledge and expertise, technologies, therapies, and other forms of exchange" between the aid apparatus and its respective clients and donors (2010, 85). James's separation of these two economies allows her to closely follow specific actors and institutions involved in both. Her work is also particularly attentive to specifically Haitian modes of subjectivity and inter-subjectivity, including those shaped by Vodou.[1]

In choosing to work within a broader moral economy framework, I intend both to articulate the term as a means of gaining deeper understanding of specific ethnographic data and to contribute to the development of the concept more broadly, increasing its relevance for anthropological analysis. For the purposes of this text, I define a moral economy as a system of transfers, exchanges, valuations, and calculations governed by notions of right, wrong, good, and evil.[2] The use of the term *system* presupposes a demarcation of phenomena that fall within and outside of a particular analysis, one that will vary according to research orientations. Using the term in its singular rather than plural form further accentuates the anthropologist's role in delineating the parameters of his or her analysis; there are no a priori criteria for determining what falls within or outside of a particular moral economy. While Fassin calls for analyzing "tensions and conflicts *between* different moral economies in order to analyze their stakes" (2009, 1266, emphasis added), my research illustrates the results of examining specific convergences and divergences *within* a moral economy, including shared objectives, contested definitions, and mutual appraisals. This approach also allows me to demonstrate how two phenomena that are treated as discrete processes—international medical aid and the emigration of health professionals—are intimately connected in the Haitian context.[3] Analytical tools that consider flows and movements of people, goods, and representations are particularly essential to studies of the Caribbean region, whose history and present are marked by the legacies of European and North American colonialism and imperialism, the transatlantic slave trade, and the various migrations of laborers, merchants, tourists, and aid workers.

During my research with Haitian and expatriate health professionals, it became apparent that a moral economy approach could bring into relief the ways that individuals involved in both international medical aid and projects to emigrate consistently interpret others' actions and intentions and are aware (in varying degrees) of their appraisal by others. The three components I use to articulate this moral economy—interest, credit, and debt—provide not only tools for comprehending the specificities of the Haitian case but also conceptual categories for comparing this context with others and identifying some of the more widespread patterns in contemporary global health interventions. This approach is not simply about finding Haitian equivalents of English-language economic terms (although English, French, and Haitian Creole's shared Latin roots do lead to a significant number of cognates). Rather, it serves to illustrate how the moral-economic concerns expressed by my informants are grouped around particular nodes. By extension, it also illustrates that taken-for-granted divisions of morality and economics into discrete realms are traced differently or may disappear altogether depending on the context in question.

Interest

In each of the three languages that predominate in Haiti's transnational aid and medical landscapes, interest has multiple meanings that carry both positive and negative connotations. In conventional economic terms, interest refers to the fee paid for borrowed assets. Certain forms of interest (also referred to as usury when considered excessive) have been condemned in a wide range of religious and ethical traditions (Lewison 1999; Mews and Abraham 2007), but it remains a central component of capitalist economies. In its more positive manifestations, interest can also refer to a benefit or an advantage, a stake or a share, or curiosity about or attention to something. All of these dimensions of the term were present in my informants' discussions of international aid.

During interviews and discussions, the foreign health workers and volunteers I spoke with rarely addressed their own interests in carrying out health interventions in Haiti using explicit terms. As Alex de Waal (1997, 4) notes, humanitarianism is self-justifying, which may preclude its proponents' need to explain their actions. I occasionally heard statements such as "I've been so fortunate in my life, and I wanted to do something to help others," but more often informants responded to my questions about how and why they began their activities in Haiti by describing the individuals or organizations that facilitated their first trips rather than the reasons for their involvement. North American clinicians, especially those on short-term trips, were particularly likely to focus on the immediate sensations associated with their activities, including the satisfaction of seeing patients they had helped and the pleasure of reconnecting and working with Haitian colleagues and partners. More than one volunteer described activities in Haiti as being "addictive" or talked about the processes through which they became "hooked." One US hospital technician laughingly told me that her passion for volunteering in Haiti resulted from "brain chemistry."

Even if foreign aid workers rarely articulated the interests that compelled their actions, these became apparent through my observations and interactions over time. They included the desire to help others, the opportunity to travel and learn, career advancement, the desire for prominence and recognition, a way of assuaging guilt, sentiments of attachment to Haiti or the Haitian population, and the pursuit of ideals such as social justice and global health. Interests and the transactions they generate in finance economies can reflect many desires and objectives, serve many purposes, and defy reductionist explanations. Similarly, interests in a moral economy can be multiple and, at times, contradictory.

The fact that these interests were rarely made explicit by the foreign clinicians, however, contributed to their becoming the subjects of conjecture by other participants in this moral economy. Haitian health professionals had questions and doubts about foreigners' interests in carrying out medical aid. Some simply stated their uncertainty: "I don't know why they come here." However, most of my Haitian informants spoke in terms that, while avoiding outright condemnation, expressed concerns over hidden interests: "I wonder about their *real* reasons for coming to Haiti." At times, Haitian health professionals linked individuals' activities to larger institutional or governmental interests, such as the commonly repeated assumption that foreign clinicians' preoccupations with reducing HIV/AIDS rates in Haiti were in fact manifestations of the interests of their respective governments in protecting the health of their own populations. It was not unusual for informants to frame their suspicions in binary terms: "Some come because they really want to help, others are here for the wrong reasons"; "I can't tell you if it's because they love Haiti, or because they were hired to do this work." The Haitian health workers I interviewed named a host of morally suspect interests that drew foreigners to their country: to be seen doing good, to experience rare and dramatic pathologies, to benefit from tax credits from their own governments, or to try out experimental medical procedures on Haitian patients. Oftentimes, they were able to give specific examples of cases they had witnessed or heard about that confirmed their suspicions.[4] One category of interests was not a subject of speculation but simply accepted as an obvious fact: the higher salaries and more comfortable living conditions associated with working in the international aid sector, specifically larger institutions such as governmental agencies or major NGOs.

This association is made despite the diversity in forms of aid. The higher salaries, comparatively luxurious living conditions, and access to significant resources of many international aid workers in Port-au-Prince are apparent to people throughout Haiti, particularly to professionals, who have often studied and lived in the capital. While this is less the case in secondary cities and rural areas, even overseas volunteers who pay for their travel to Haiti and may live in what they consider to be rudimentary conditions (sleeping on military cots, not having access to hot water, eating a homogeneous diet, etc.) enjoy resources during their stay that are unavailable to the majority of Haitians: private transportation, sufficient food, safe housing and water supplies, and, above all, the possibility of returning home to a wealthy country.

While many foreign clinicians in Haiti do not receive salaried remuneration for their services, there exists a wide range of arrangements related to stipends, per diems, and benefits that Haitians identify as potential interests for their colleagues from overseas. For example, Cuban health workers in Haiti receive free housing and a monthly stipend of 300 USD that dwarfs their regular Cuban salary of approximately 27 USD per month. I was told by both Cuban and Haitian informants that serving as an *internacionalista* can improve working conditions upon returning to Cuba, particularly with regard to assignment in urban areas, which are considered more desirable in terms of their proximity to various resources and opportunities. Finally, missions to countries such as Haiti allow for the opportunity to purchase household appliances such as stoves, refrigerators, and computers, items that are difficult to obtain in Cuba. While it would be unjustified to argue that the officially stated interests of solidarity with the Haitian people have no importance for individual Cuban clinicians, it would be similarly unwarranted to dismiss the pragmatic concerns that make missions to Haiti interesting in other ways.

One reason that these tangible interests are so apparent to Haitian health care workers as they observe their foreign counterparts is that they are particularly relevant to their own lives. While earning significantly more than the majority of their fellow citizens, most Haitian health professionals live in a context of resource scarcity, and economic concerns predominate when they talk of emigration and professional futures. For example, at the time I interviewed them, Haitian medical residents were earning 200 USD a month for full-time work and were forbidden to engage in other salaried employment. Some of the medical residents already had children, many others planned to have them in the future, and all were expected to eventually help support aging parents and other family members. Not only was their salary insufficient to cover what they considered to be their basic immediate needs but their paychecks were also delayed for many months, forcing them to borrow money from relatives and friends. Young Haitian physicians are well aware that even working for NGOs or in private clinics is far less lucrative than employment abroad. One told me, "My friend from medical school just got a residency in Miami. He's earning $80,000 a year! How could I ever earn that in Haiti?" In contemplating their professional and personal interests, young Haitian physicians (and young professionals in other fields) were most likely to be looking for opportunities outside their country.

Fully cognizant of the lack of health professionals throughout Haiti and its impact on their country's population, young Haitian clinicians were confronted with a contradiction between their own interests and those of their nation. In all spheres of life, it is common to hear people in Haiti complain about *enterè pèsonèl* (personal interest), stakes held by individuals that were the downfall of collective initiatives and social projects. Personal interest, for example, could be blamed for mismanaged, wasted, or diverted resources in the health sector. Informants gave examples of unscrupulous aid intermediaries who sold donated medication in their private pharmacies or who allotted a scholarship for medical study abroad to a relative rather than to a more deserving candidate. Personal interest was often identified as the source of the country's many problems, from economic ruin to political instability and environmental degradation.[5]

In describing their plans for emigration, my Haitian informants often framed the decision in personal terms, describing poor living conditions, a lack of opportunities for professional development, and various kinds of insecurity as *pa enteresan* (not interesting). But they also tended to frame the interests more broadly, most often referring to family: "I want my children to go to good schools"; "I want to be able to help my parents by sending money back for them to build a decent house." Some, citing the example of successful health and social projects initiated by members of the Haitian diaspora, pointed to emigration as the best way to "do something for my country." While it would be easy to attribute this framing of interests as a means of self-justification or deflecting criticism, the tragic and prevailing sentiment expressed by many Haitians that their country does not have a viable future (Beckett 2008) carries with it the implication that their most promising interests lie elsewhere.

The high rate of emigration of health professionals from Haiti and from other impoverished settings has emerged as a growing concern for global health leaders and organizations. While earlier configurations of international medical intervention focused on containing the spread of infectious diseases or eliminating specific pathologies, an increasing number of initiatives focus on strengthening health systems and evaluating interventions in terms of their sustainability, a goal that is premised on the nonemigration of health workers. With the increased attention placed on training and retaining local health professionals, varied and contradictory interests emerge and become a source of tensions.

Actors in a moral economy scrutinize each other's interests, trying both to determine who is working to what ends and to prove that their own interests are legitimate and morally acceptable. Questions about interests are more often asked than answered. Does a Cuban physician volunteer to work in Haiti in order to express solidarity with the population of a neighboring country or in order to increase her chances of working in Havana upon returning to Cuba? What does a Canadian physician appreciate more: the gratitude expressed by patients in a rural Haitian village or the accolades he receives from his colleagues back home? Framing the questions in these terms presupposes that interests are necessarily hierarchical and mutually exclusive. They also signal that the person asking the question is savvy enough not to be duped by the illusion of disinterested aid. It seems, however, that some hopes remain for generous altruism or beneficent interests; otherwise the exposés of morally suspect interests and corruption would have ceased to enjoy their current traction and visibility. Despite my Haitian informants' general skepticism about the interests of expatriate aid workers in their country, I frequently heard references to altruistic foreigners who had been *des vrais amis d'Haïti* (true friends of Haiti). This was most often in reference to individuals who had passed away but left some tangible and enduring legacy—for example, a clinic or an irrigation system—and informants often stressed the indiscriminate nature of the aid: "She helped anyone who needed it, no matter who they were."

Not only does an attention to interest stay close to the language of my informants but it also allows for a consideration of both affective and material factors that shape action and perceptions. Motivation is often used to explain behaviors but is more likely to be understood in individualized and internalized terms. In addition, interest better reflects the temporality associated with my informants' aspirations and suspicions. Like interest in conventional economics, interests in a moral economy may grow or diminish over time, leading to desirable or undesirable outcomes and always offering the promise or threat of change. Actions that serve others' interests rather than one's own are also a means for accruing credit, a second component in this moral economy.

Credit

Anthropologists theorizing about credit have placed it in a dyad with debt and link the two to temporality, to power, and to morality. Without using the term *moral economy*, Gustav Peebles (2010) argues for a continued juxtaposition of the moral and economic dimensions of credit and debt, and details the contribution of ethnographic work on the topic. In the Haitian context, *kredi* is often mentioned as something a store or business will not extend. "Pa mande kredi!" (Don't ask for credit!), warn handwritten signs in shops. Monetary *credit* is based on an act of recognition, and the term is used in Haitian Creole as in English to describe recognition accorded to a deserving party: "Bay li kredi pou sa li fè" (Give her credit for what she did). Haitians also use the verb *rekonèt* (recognize), which like its English counterpart carries the connotation of acknowledgment. The noun *rekonesans*, tellingly, translates as gratitude.

Perhaps the most obvious dimension of credit in the realm of international health interventions is the recognition of one's actions: *who gets credit for* an act or an intervention. This recognition can be afforded by the recipient in the form of verbal thanks, countergifts, and other expressions of individual gratitude, but credit can also be solicited from and afforded by a larger audience. The media for accruing credit vary but often involve visual manifestations. Large placards describing a government-sponsored aid project, an individual's name printed on a plaque or stenciled directly onto a donated building, and boxes of donations marked with logos or flags: these means of claiming a current intervention also serve to establish *credibility* for future projects. This credibility may help attract additional resources, form new alliances, and defend against impending threats. Credit in this arena is frequently attributed through visual ascriptions, including names and logos painted on walls, commemorative plaques, and slogans emblazoned on T-shirts. In some instances, elaborate ceremonies—involving speeches, prayers, processions, dance, theater, and songs—both mark the opening of a new clinic or the graduation of a cohort of medical or nursing students and provide an opportunity to publicly identify the actors who contributed to the event's raison d'être.

Not receiving credit for one's work in this context is often a source of acrimony. In the case of young Haitian physicians, many expressed their frustration at not having their deeds valued or acknowledged, while foreign medical workers or volunteers often benefited from visibility, recognition, and access to resources. Who gets credit for medical aid is often a contentious issue, as participants' roles are varied and the diverse resources they contribute are often not commensurable. For example, a Canadian nurse might receive thanks for bringing donated pharmaceuticals to Haiti, but her Haitian counterpart, after spending hours counting, bagging, and dispensing the medication, may have her efforts go unrecognized. Not getting credit for their efforts or perceived sacrifices was frequently named by medical residents as a factor motivating their desire to emigrate. As described in the previous chapter, when the residents in Cap-Haïtien went on strike in 2008, a recurring theme in their chants, posters, and speeches was the common Haitian proverb "Bourik travay, chwal galonnen" (The donkey works, the horse gets the honors).

The acrimony that results from its nonattribution signals the importance of credit as a resource, one that may not be immediately expended but can be stored for use at a later time. Individuals and organizations can earn credit through visible and successful projects that facilitate future interventions. A sustained and long-term presence (particularly in a context where a large number of bodies are competing for attention and resources) is used as credit: endurance and consistency help make one a desirable recipient. Assigning credibility through previous actions became particularly salient after the 2010 earthquake, when a high number of individuals and groups new to Haiti competed with existing actors for attention, donations, and other resources. A Cuban writer described his country's contribution in these terms: "Aid from Cuba to the people of Haiti did not come with the earthquake. Cuba has developed an Integrated Health Plan in Haiti since 1998, in which over 6,000 Cuban health workers have participated"

(Manzaneda 2010). It is common for groups to describe themselves (or to be described by others) in terms of duration of involvement and scope of accomplishment, both of which allow credit to accumulate in order to establish a position of moral reliability and act as a lever of potential further support. However, this tendency can be a double-edged sword, with critics of aid highlighting the persistence of abysmal health and social conditions in Haiti in spite of—or as a result of—the enduring and pervasive presence of foreign interventions.

I also encountered situations in which individuals and groups did not want to receive credit for their actions. One such occasion involved Konbit Sante. After extensive consultation with ministry staff and local health leaders, the organization applied for and received a grant from a US foundation to build a pediatric emergency room at the HUJ. When I spoke with Konbit Sante's director Nate Nickerson the day before the room's inauguration ceremony, he was distressed by a news report about the event that he had just heard on a local radio station. The announcer had named Konbit Sante several times, giving the group credit for creating this valuable new service. Nickerson gave two reasons for his discontent. By giving credit to the NGO, the radio announcer had undermined the organization's explicit goals of working to strengthen the public health sector and increase the credibility of the Haitian state in the eyes of the population. In addition, Nickerson voiced a more pragmatic concern: he knew from prior experiences that when the organization's name received this sort of visibility, it increased the number of appeals for aid from other individuals and organizations in the community, most of which he would have to turn down because of limited resources.

Drawing on this episode, we can also see how individuals other than executors may have stakes in how credit is attributed. After the pediatric emergency room was inaugurated, hospital administrators insisted that Konbit Sante's logo be prominently painted above the main entrance. Nickerson protested, emphasizing that the creation of the unit had been a collaborative effort and that the Haitian government and hospital leadership had played an equally important part in bringing the project to fruition. I heard from hospital staff, however, that in cases where it was perceived by the local population that an intervention would not have taken place without private, foreign, or nongovernmental support, it was important that the latter clearly receive credit for their interventions. This was in part to preclude the Haitian government's claiming or receiving credit where it was not due. For nearly all of my Haitian informants, the Haitian state had not fulfilled its obligations to its citizenry, particularly in the areas of health care and public services. In their eyes, this failure also led the state to take credit for others' actions, in what were perceived to be immoral attempts at self-legitimization and self-justification.

The attribution of credit, therefore, must be understood not as a simple consequence of valued actions, but rather as a socially mediated process that generates tensions and struggles. Getting credit for one's actions in a moral economy is more than a matter of simple visibility; it also acts as a platform for prominence in spheres where actors, organizations, and institutions vie for resources. The means for accumulating credit in the context I have discussed range from proficiency in the forms of accountability that fall within the scope of "audit culture" (Strathern 2000) to the visibility and charisma of individuals who are considered to be effective and morally reliable conduits between donors and recipients.

Debt

Debt, according to David Graeber, "is just an exchange that has not been brought to completion" (2011, 121). Like the two components just discussed, debt can be framed in national, institutional, and individual terms. Analysts have often blamed Haiti's financial debts to other nations and global financial institutions for the country's poverty and its effects on Haitians' health (Farmer 1992, 2001). A series of recent debt cancellation measures by international financial bodies was hailed by many as an important step toward improving economic conditions in Haiti (International Monetary Fund 2009), and the US Congress passed Haiti-specific debt relief in 2011. Converse debts framed in national terms involve foreign nations' debts to Haiti—specifically those directly connected to the country's past—and involve historical events with both specific material consequences and powerful symbolic valence. Foremost among them are France's debt to Haiti for its colonial legacy of slavery and exploitation and for the enormous sum—calculated at more than 20 billion USD—it extorted from Haiti's postrevolutionary government as compensation for damage to French property, including enslaved persons and plantations.[6] The United States' debt to Haiti is invoked by Haitians (and a small number of US scholars and activists) for the latter's assistance during the American Revolution as well as in discussions of wrongs committed during the twentieth century, including the military occupation from 1915 to 1934, support for the Duvalier dictatorship, and policy undermining democratic movements and popular sovereignty in the last three decades.[7] Finally, Haiti's support for nineteenth-century Latin American independence movements and hospitality toward Simón Bolívar are often invoked in terms of debts in contemporary discourse on Latin American nations' aid to Haiti (Telesur 2011).

While these nationalist framings of debt appeared in official discourses or in rhetorical reflections on Haiti's international relations, individuals' negotiation of debt was more often expressed in terms of giving back. For members of the Haitian diaspora who had returned to participate in medical projects, this formulation was relatively straightforward: they had benefited from the resources of their homeland, whether through tangible resources and opportunities or a sense of self, identity, and national pride, and they felt compelled or obligated to *remèt* (return or give back) to their country through services to those remaining in Haiti. The Haitian American and Haitian Canadian clinicians I interviewed framed these debts using strong nationalist, patriotic, and affective terms, speaking of *la patrie* (the homeland), *lakay* (home), or *Ayiti, manman cheri* (Haiti, dear mother).[8]

These sentiments, however, had not developed among the hopeful emigrants I interviewed. Rather than speak of their debts toward Haiti, it was much more common for young Haitian physicians to identify the ways in which their country, specifically its leaders and elite, had taken advantage of their youth and talents, exploiting them without offering any promises of future rewards. Their state owed them, not only for the salaries that were subject to months of delay but also for its destructive patterns of neglect, exploitation, and corruption. Their relationship to the Haitian population at large was addressed in more ambivalent terms. Some stated that patients had no respect or gratitude for them (particularly in their position as young doctors), while others described patients who treated them with deference and affection. One young physician told me that she wanted to stay in Haiti simply because the slightest gesture she made for her patients—a kind word, medical advice, or the most basic treatment—was met with such gratitude. While the residents I interviewed did not interpret their clinical activities at that time as a way of paying a debt, it seems likely that they may eventually adopt the framing used by emigrants after their own departure.

For North American clinicians who used the expression "giving back" to describe their work in Haiti, the debt or countergift was directed toward an unspecified recipient. Although Haiti as a national entity and the Haitian population represented objects of affection for many of them, they did not voice the nationalist sentiments expressed by clinicians from the diaspora. The expression "giving back" implies a dyad; however, the American and Canadian clinicians who use it do not imply that they are engaging in an exchange with a specific gift partner. Rather, they frame their activities in terms of a generalized reciprocity, all the while knowing that they are unlikely to ever need the type of services they usually dispense in Haiti—namely, primary health care resulting from extreme poverty and lack of infrastructure.[9] When I questioned them further about the phrase, those who used it clarified that they conceived of their work as a redistribution of resources that they had received in excess because of factors beyond their control, including their place of birth. This framing of international aid activities as redistribution was echoed in the discourses of Haitian health workers, whom I never heard describe foreign clinicians' activities in their country as a form of debt.

In classic gift theories, debts resulting from gifts must be repaid with countergifts (Mauss 1950). If one chooses to view international medical aid to Haiti as a form of gift, countergifts from Haitian health professionals who receive or channel aid are often absent. Both Haitian and foreign informants mentioned the discomfort that resulted when, after a provision of aid in some form, recipients requested further assistance. Some foreign clinicians responded by framing a propensity for dependence and solicitation as an innate Haitian quality; conversely, some Haitian clinicians criticized the amount of aid disbursed as so paltry or flawed that it revealed the intent by foreigners and their governments to keep Haiti in a state of dependence. Debts and gifts are not the only lens through which international medical interventions can be examined; however, my research indicates that these framings and the tensions associated with them have particular salience in the Haitian setting.

Like interest and credit, evaluations around debts are subject to controversy. On a national and global scale, these are apparent in debates concerning reparations for colonial exploitation and slavery, the relevance of which is particularly obvious in Haiti. While my informants uniformly expressed a sentiment of injustice in terms of their nation's relations with more powerful states, a desire to rectify this injustice through reparations or the settling of debts was tempered by a desire to end foreign interventions in Haiti's affairs and, most important, the hope for national autonomy and self-determination. At the same time, the current configurations of global capitalism and geopolitics made any condition resembling national sovereignty difficult, if not impossible, to envision.

Beyond Haiti

Medicine, humanitarianism, and transnational relations in Haiti are realms that are frequently experienced, negotiated, and represented in terms of calculations, transfers, exchanges, and morality. Morality and economics, which are difficult to distinguish in any setting, are particularly inextricable in settings of marked inequalities in resources. The three components I have described in this chapter, in addition to being conventional economic terms, can also be studied as morally saturated categories. Thinking about these concepts in terms of a moral economy draws attention to the collective and shared nature of efforts that mobilize, enable, and respond to international aid. Both morality and economics always surpass individual and subjective experiences to encompass broader relations and social networks, even if in so doing they engender clashes in individuals' perspectives and claims. They are also well suited for analyses in light of the mobility and fluidity that have long characterized the Caribbean region and that are now recognized as inherent to a postcolonial, globalized world.

The presence of international influences through its health system is not unique to Haiti, and work elsewhere on humanitarian and global health interventions (particularly in Africa; see Redfield 2005, Brada 2010, and Wendland 2010) confirms that particular patterns and trends are occurring on a much larger scale, albeit with local specificities. A moral economy approach highlights the inextricability of two phenomena that are often considered separately in development and policy circles: the provision of health services by expatriate clinicians in impoverished settings and the emigration of health professionals from these settings to aid-sending countries. At first glance, the links between the two phenomena appear more purely economic and technical. The professional employees of international organizations and agencies often have access to the increased salaries, linguistic capital, and transnational networks that facilitate emigration processes. But thinking with the components of a moral economy described earlier sheds light on less visible ties and tensions between the two phenomena. Young Haitian clinicians see their interests—whether for professional development, a higher quality of life, or opportunities to contribute to their country's economy—as lying abroad, while foreign aid groups' interests in strengthening Haiti's health care system are increasingly contingent on the nonemigration of Haitian professionals. While Haitian clinicians assert that not receiving recognition for their efforts is an important factor in fueling their departure, foreign aid workers, volunteers, and students continue to receive various forms of credit (salaries, admiration, academic credit in global health courses and training programs) for their work in Haiti. Finally, aid and emigration are both responses to and instigators of various types of debt, ranging from remittances to the relatives who contributed to visa fees and a plane ticket to Miami to the care of strangers as a form of giving back one's good fortune.

This effort to promote the use of a moral economy as an analytic tool and to offer a means for refining what has been an alluring yet elusive concept reflects my agreement with Fassin that a moral economy is indeed a "concept in becoming." My goal in this analysis is not simply to find ethnographic examples of the commonplace economic concepts used in industrialized settings. Rather, it emerged from the desire to work with concepts whose components ("moral" and "economy") apply to such a limitless diversity of referents that scholars are often confronted with the proverbial "sledgehammer to crack a nut" idiom. This becomes even more evident when we consider that all economies have moral dimensions and all moralities have economic dimensions. Articulating a moral economy in terms of its components offers a way of creating surfaces of engagement with ethnographic material, one that illustrates the many ways in which participants enact and gauge a range of encounters, exchanges, and calculations. Working in the framework of ethnography as theory (Nader 2011), this approach helps ensure that the analytic tools we develop to describe processes and affects allow for comparisons across time and locality while remaining grounded in the lives and realities of individuals and communities.

SAINTS, VILLAINS, AND CHAMPIONS

"What I've come to realize," Estelle told me, "is that a lot of the donors don't seem to care that much about what the organization is doing in the community, about our partners and the staff in Haiti. It seems like they're supporting the organization because of *me*, because *I'm* the director!" Estelle was not only surprised by this realization but she also found it distressing and burdensome. As a member of one of Haiti's most politically and economically prominent families, Estelle came to the United States as a young adult in the late 1950s, fleeing the threat of François Duvalier's violent dictatorship. She returned to Haiti over three decades later and cofounded a small organization that works to improve health conditions in a rural area. Today, the organization supports a hospital, mobile clinics, and diverse community development initiatives. While a number of institutions and individuals in the United States support the projects as donors and volunteers, Estelle is the driving force and public face of the organization.

Estelle's story is one with an appealing narrative arc: she is not only an immigrant who remembered her roots and has devoted much of her adult life to supporting her homeland but also someone who crossed boundaries of class and color to work in a community very different from the one she came from. As a long-term US citizen and resident, her demeanor and modes of communication are familiar to American donors and supporters; as a Haitian, she also embodies a "native's" knowledge of and commitment to her country of origin.

Paradoxically, Estelle also represents one of the most vilified categories of individuals in the world of transnational aid and humanitarianism: a member of the privileged, elite class of poorer nations. In the context of Haiti, this class is sometimes described in expatriate circles and academic texts as MREs ("Morally Repugnant Elites" or "Most Repugnant Elites"). They are accused of causing or participating in the country's deterioration through economic exploitation, repressive governance, and excluding Haiti's majority from participation in civic life. Not only in Haiti but also in countries around the world where European colonialism and slavery created and reinforced hierarchies and inequalities, one finds systems of racial and color stratification that favor white, European traits. In the United States, Estelle told me that she was sometimes asked if she was Turkish or North African. In the Haitian village where she worked, people who did not know her usually mistook her for a *blan*. Although she was able to laugh at some of the situations that resulted from these assumptions (for example, having people who were talking about her presume that she would not understand them), it also caused her frustration and pain. "Kiyès ki blan?" (Who's a foreigner?) I remember her yelling at a group of teenagers who referred to her using the term, her voice shaking.

In her efforts to move resources from the world's wealthiest countries to one of the world's poorest, Estelle had to confront the expectations that the diverse actors involved in the aid process (recipients, donors, implementers) had of her. These expectations are often structured according to a set of archetypal figures that shape existing narratives of aid and have tangible impacts on how interventions are designed and implemented.

In this chapter, I will focus on three such figures—namely, saints, villains, and champions. For each figure, I will draw from the experiences and representations of specific individuals, as well as from common tropes about these categories that circulate in depictions of and discussions about aid. It is important to keep in mind that, while saints, champions, and villains exist as distinct archetypes, specific individuals can occupy more than one these categories, depending on who is doing the classification. Inclusion in any one of these groups is not necessarily stable or secure. One can fall from being a saint to a villain, or conversely, experience the opposite process through redemptive transformation.

Through these discussions, I hope to complement a large body of work on what is probably the most visible archetypical figure in depictions of humanitarianism, that of the victim. Victims are embodied by a number of categories: the patient, the refugee, the woman, and most quintessentially, the child. They are akin to what Leslie Butt (2002) called the "suffering stranger" in her early critique of how individuals were represented by academics writing about health and social justice. Joel Robbins (2013) argued that representations of "suffering subjects" replaced those of "primitive others" starting in the 1990s. My decision not to address victims here stems both from the extensive attention the category has received from other authors (Bornstein 2010; Malkki 2010, 2015; Dahl 2015), and my concern throughout this book with the providers and intermediaries of medical aid. While my discussion of the saint figure will be the most extensive, the figures of the villain and champion allow us to move beyond the reductive binary of donors and recipients that often characterizes descriptions of humanitarian encounters.

My discussion of the saint figure will focus on the humanitarian doctor as exemplified by the physician-anthropologist Paul Farmer. Farmer has been described by the *New York Times* columnist Nicholas Kristof as "pretty much a saint" and by Jeffrey Sachs as "a saint of global health." He spent many years working in Haiti's Central Plateau, and the organization he cofounded, Partners in Health (PIH) and its Haitian counterpart Zanmi Lasante (ZL) have become major figures in providing health services in a growing number of communities in central Haiti. PIH/ZL has become the second largest provider of health services in Haiti after the government of Haiti, and the group's flagship hospital, the Hôpital Universitaire de Mirebalais, is now the country's second largest hospital.

Farmer was an extraordinary example, in terms of his capacities as an individual, his visibility and reputation on an international scale, and the impact his work has had on individuals, populations, and health systems. A close examination of his life and work not only provides information about key actors in Haiti's health sector but also affords insight into the place of charismatic individuals in transnational health interventions, and context for debates around "white saviors" and neocolonialism in global health. Finally, analyzing the work of Farmer (and other saintly figures such as the Alsatian physician Albert Schweitzer, renowned for the hospital he founded in Lambaréné, in what is now Gabon) sheds light on the emergence of secular humanitarianism in Europe and North America in the twentieth and twenty-first centuries. Although contemporary humanitarianism has been profoundly influenced by Judeo-Christian traditions, many aid workers explicitly renounce faith-based or missionary initiatives. However, the figure of the Christian saint continues to occupy a central place in medical aid and global health projects and programs, even though aid workers themselves may express discomfort with such a figure, or even disavow it (Malkki 2015, 26–30).

In the years I have been conducting research on medical aid in Haiti, I have been struck by the two ways that North American colleagues in anthropology, public health, and medicine have spoken to me about Farmer's work. The majority speak in admiring terms. They are impressed by Farmer's scholarship and inspired by his commitment to improving the health conditions of impoverished populations. A smaller but not unsubstantial group has expressed critical perspectives, asking (sometimes hopefully) if my own research identifies any negative aspects of Farmer's activities in Haiti. I suspect that there are different factors motivating the desire to see such an influential figure unmasked or exposed. One of these may be professional jealousy. Farmer was without a doubt one of the world's most renowned and influential anthropologists and physicians. Another factor could be the desire for an "Icarian" arc to Farmer's story. Research on narrative form has shown that a rising then falling tendency is among the most common story arcs (Reagan et al. 2016). As I stated in the introduction to this book, I have no desire to write an exposé of international aid in Haiti, nor of Farmer or the organizations he founded and worked with. I have a deep admiration for his scholarship (in particular his early works), for his commitment to the people of Haiti, and for PIH/ZL's successes in increasing health care (including access to lifesaving medications) to millions of people who would not have benefited from it otherwise.

My preoccupations as an anthropologist do not revolve around Farmer's moral worth or qualities as an individual, or around the strengths and weaknesses of his interventions in Haiti. I am in no position to evaluate these, having only briefly met him twice during public lectures and having visited one of PIH/ZL's clinical sites on a single occasion.[1] The organizations are not active in northern Haiti where I conducted my research. In the preceding pages, I have presented descriptions and analyses of medical aid and Haitian health professionals in ways that I intend as complementary to Farmer's work on the political economy of health and structural violence. In addition, by thinking through Farmer's place and influence in the emergence of contemporary global health, I provide insights into why charismatic individuals from privileged backgrounds occupy such a central place in models and aspirations for positive social change, as opposed to movements based on collective action, shifts in political and economic governance, and initiatives advanced by those belonging to subaltern populations. Considerations of how racial dynamics play out in humanitarian encounters have led to critiques of "white savior" dynamics in global health. Why have these individuals tended to be white, male physicians, and how does this legacy persist in contemporary global health interventions? How do characterizations of saints (and other archetypical figures) shape the provision of health services in impoverished settings, influencing everything from the types of services provided to expectations about what is appropriate behavior by the actors involved in medical encounters? In the first chapter of this book, I noted that many foreign aid organizations operating in Haiti tend to have charismatic leaders, and that this model of governance can make the coordination of interventions challenging. In the following sections, I will demonstrate that membership in and distance from groups of "suffering strangers" are paramount in evaluations of who is hailed or reviled in aid encounters.

"From Harvard to Haiti"

While Farmer did not write extensively about his own life, Tracy Kidder's 2003 biography, *Mountains beyond Mountains: The Quest of Dr. Paul Farmer, a Man Who Would Cure the World*, provides a thorough coverage of Farmer's background and life trajectory. Born in 1959 to working-class parents in Massachusetts, Farmer grew up in Alabama and Florida, where his family resided for extended periods in a school bus and on a boat. Kidder's recounting depicts a childhood of success in school, early exposure to literature, and few material comforts. Farmer first traveled to Haiti in 1983, having met Haitian migrant workers through progressive Catholic communities while an undergraduate at Duke University. He continued to travel to Haiti during his years of graduate study at Harvard University, where he earned both a medical degree and a doctorate in anthropology. (Farmer would go on to become a professor at Harvard, and chaired the Department of Global Health and Social Medicine at Harvard Medical School.) The late 1980s were a particularly tumultuous period in Haiti, with the fall of the thirty-year Duvalier dictatorship in 1986 and a string of provisional governments and military coups in the years that followed. Along with Episcopal church leaders and other international students and volunteers, Farmer established a clinic in the rural settlement of Cange, and eventually cofounded PIH/ZL, the groups that would come to structure and support the clinic and other health initiatives. In the years that followed, PIH developed similar programs by founding organizations in Peru, Russia, and seven other countries. The organization has also worked in Massachusetts and the Navajo Nation. Since 2005 Farmer had been particularly active in Rwanda where he worked with PIH and its Rwandan counterpart, Inshuti Mu Buzima, and in West Africa since 2014, following the devastating Ebola outbreak in that region. A 2017 documentary, *Bending the Arc*, traced Farmer's trajectory, along with that of his PIH cofounders Jim-Yong Kim and Ophelia Dahl, and notable colleagues such as the Rwandan physician Agnes Binagwaho.

Farmer's earliest anthropological research drew from classic approaches in comparative ethnomedicine while critiquing the limitations of these same approaches. He described the ailments of *move san* (bad blood) and *lèt gate* (spoiled milk) among rural Haitian women, using the framework of "explanatory models" to show the contrast between the afflicted women's and local healers' understanding of the conditions as being rooted in malignant emotions and those of biomedical doctors who dismissed the ailments. He concluded that existing models of folk illness, somatization, or Western psychiatric categories are inadequate for understanding conditions such as *move san* and *lèt gate*, and instead highlighted the need for an "anthropology of suffering" (Farmer 1988). In later works, Farmer drew from several theoretical models, including Johan Galtung's

concept of structural violence in order to illustrate the pernicious effects of poverty and inequalities on populations, as well as world systems theories developed
by scholars such as Immanuel Wallerstein and Sidney Mintz to trace the effects of
global commerce, neoliberal economic policies, and international development
projects on the health of individuals living in what seem to be remote areas that
are cut off from the rest of the world. His 1992 monograph *AIDS and Accusation:
Haiti and the Geography of Blame* examined the arrival of HIV/AIDS in Haiti's
Central Plateau, and includes analyses of both local responses to the virus as well
as the ways in which Americans' association of the diseases with Haiti was a con-
tinuation of centuries of prejudice and stigma against the country and its people. Farmer also drew from liberation theology in his work, specifically from the
endeavor to understand the forces of oppression in order to overthrow them. In
Infections and Inequalities (1999) and *Pathologies of Power* (2003), Farmer developed his analyses of how poverty, inequality, and injustice contribute to sickness
and suffering around the world. His more recent books include an account of
the 2010 earthquake and its aftermath in Haiti (2011) and *Fevers, Feuds and Diamonds: Ebola and the Ravages of History* (2020), which situates narratives of Ebola
survivors within the larger context of colonialism and violence in West Africa.

Throughout his writings and in his public speaking engagements, Farmer
described the illnesses of individuals he had encountered or treated as a clinician. Narratives from Haiti were predominant in his early works. These included
a young woman whose family was displaced by the construction of an American-
designed hydroelectric dam—the family's ensuing poverty forced her to seek out
domestic work in the capital city of Port-au-Prince and led her to enter a sexual
relationship with a man from whom she contracted HIV. Another case is that of
a young man whose complaints about the conditions of local roads were interpreted as antigovernment sentiment during a period of military rule. As a consequence, he was beaten and tortured, and died of his wounds shortly after. Farmer
makes a convincing point: virtually any case of suffering or illness in Haiti can be
understood as a consequence of poverty, the legacies of slavery and colonialism,
and continued exploitation by international forces and Haiti's governing elite.

In his later writings, the case of Haiti was often used to illustrate Farmer's
claims and arguments related to the provision of health services. One of Farmer's
most vehement arguments is against the notion that health care for the poor
must be cost-effective. He claims, "A human rights approach to health economics and health policy helps to bring into relief the ill effects of the efficacy-equity
trade-off: this is, only if unnecessary sickness and premature death don't matter
can inegalitarian systems ever be considered efficacious" (Farmer 2003, 19). The
struggle for equity is a recurring theme in Farmer's writings and a motivating
force in his clinical activities.

Farmer's work illustrates the increasing overlap and intensified relationship between humanitarianism and human rights. Both frameworks are prominent in his work, which uses the language and logic of human rights—namely, the right to adequate health services and a decent standard of living—in what can be interpreted as a classic humanitarian project: the provision of assistance to the poor and suffering. In Farmer's case, the form of assistance (medical services) is particularly salient, as he frequently drew on his status as a physician to reinforce his claims and justify his perspectives. Doing so contributed to his goal of convincing readers of the feasibility and desirability of treating poor patients.

Farmer has been enormously influential within anthropology and medicine, and his clinical practice, research, and advocacy have attracted attention worldwide. Farmer's recognition by colleagues are particularly noteworthy. He has been awarded several major prizes by anthropological and medical societies, has received honorary doctorates from several major US universities, and is frequently invited to deliver speeches and addresses at major international events. Farmer received a MacArthur Foundation Genius Award, the Hilton Humanitarian Award, and the Berggruen Prize, and was elected to both the Institute of Medicine of the National Academy of Sciences and the American Academy of Arts and Sciences. In addition, he was named UN Special Deputy Envoy to Haiti by Bill Clinton in 2009 and UN Special Adviser to Secretary-General Ban Ki-Moon in 2012.

While Farmer had been well known among medical anthropologists and scholars of Haiti before the 2003 publication of *Mountains beyond Mountains*, Kidder's biography extended Farmer's renown to a much larger audience. The book rapidly became a national best seller, was named a Notable Book by the *New York Times*, and was taught in many schools and universities (particularly in medical schools, where it was regularly assigned as required reading for first-year students in the years after its publication). *Mountains beyond Mountains* focuses primarily on Farmer as an extraordinary individual: his brilliant intellect and photographic memory, his choice to reject material comforts and pursue a lifestyle of extraordinary self-sacrifice, and his unwavering commitment to provide health services to poor people in Haiti and other countries. Kidder describes Farmer's work in a variety of settings ranging from shacks in Peru to meetings with officials from the World Bank in Russia. Much of the book takes place in Haiti, which Farmer has called his "greatest teacher." It is in Haiti that Kidder sees many of Farmer's extraordinary traits in action—his thorough and intimate knowledge of Haitian society and history; his ability to rally resources and create a functioning health care system in an extremely impoverished and isolated area; and the tenacity of his convictions, exemplified in the following statement: "The problem is, if I don't work this hard, someone will die who doesn't have to.

That sounds megalomaniacal. I wouldn't have said that to you before I'd taken you to Haiti and you had seen that it was manifestly true" (Kidder 2003, 191). Overhearing someone refer to him as a saint, Farmer tells Kidder, "People call me a saint and I think, I have to work harder. Because a saint would be a great thing to be" (16). Of course, given Kidder's description of Farmer's lifestyle and the extreme efforts he expends to provide care and health systems for his patients, it is difficult to imagine him working any harder.

"My Doctors, My Doctors . . ."

In his own writings about Haiti, Farmer rarely addressed the existence of the hundreds of other agencies and organizations providing health care throughout Haiti. He also made fairly limited mention of MSPP and its national system of dispensaries, clinics, and hospitals. His writings instead focused on the reasons why rural Haitians are impoverished and sick, describing their lack of access to medical and other basic services, and arguing for the feasibility and necessity of providing such services. The services themselves, however, were often summarily described. The following text pertains to a PIH/ZL tuberculosis initiative:

> Those diagnosed with tuberculosis who participated in the new treat-ment program were to receive daily visits from their village health worker during the first month following diagnosis. They would also receive financial aid of thirty dollars per month for the first three months; would be eligible for nutritional supplements; would receive regular reminders from their village health worker to attend the clinic; and would receive a five-dollar honorarium to defray "travel" expenses (for example, renting a donkey) for attending the clinic. If a patient did not attend, someone from the clinic—often a physician or an auxiliary nurse—would make a visit to the no-show's house. A series of forms, including a detailed initial interview schedule and home visit reports regularized these arrangements and replaced the relatively limited forms used for other patients. (Farmer 2003, 149–50)

He goes on to describe the success of the program in curing these individuals and uses this example to argue against the prevailing view that high-quality medical services for life-threatening diseases in the context of extreme poverty are impos-sible to implement.

Given the size and scope of PIH/ZL's projects, it to be expected that they have had major impacts on communities where the group is active, particularly when one considers the paucity of health resources and infrastructure in settings like

Haiti. Once services are implemented in sites such as rural Haiti, a number of everyday complications arise: patient triage, coordination and implementation of care, hiring and retaining staff and employees, and negotiating local and national politics. In considering the tuberculosis program just described, for example, many questions emerge. Who are the village health workers and how are they selected? What relationship do they have with other individuals in the community? How is their work remunerated? What exactly happens when a physician or auxiliary nurse visits a "no-show's" house? Other anthropologists have described the conflicts and tensions between health care providers and patients in Haiti (Brodwin 1996; Maternowska 2006). It is unrealistic to imagine that such dynamics are absent from PIH/ZL's work.

Haitian health care workers rarely appear in Farmer's writings, except when mentioned as dedicated professionals and community health workers (*accompagnateurs*) employed by PIH/ZL. Excerpts from *Mountains beyond Mountains* suggest a complicated relationship between Farmer and Haitian health professionals:

> In a bed by the door of the hospital lies a moaning thirteen-year-old girl, just arrived by donkey ambulance. Two young Haitian doctors—one is just an intern—stand beside her bed, eyes half-lowered, lips pursed, as Farmer makes the Haitian hand slap, saying, "*Doktè-m yo, doktè-m yo, sa k'ap pase-n?*" [*sic*]—Doctors, doctors, what's going on with you?" His voice sounds plaintive, not angry, as he lectures: You do not administer an antibiotic to a person with meningitis until you have done a spinal tap and know the variety of meningitis and thus which drug will work. Then he does the job himself, the young doctors looking on, holding the girl down. (Kidder 2003, 32)

Kidder's translation of Farmer's admonishment is not completely accurate, as Farmer literally says "My doctors, my doctors . . ." with the possessive indicating affection, authority, or both. The climax of the anecdote is a few lines later, when Farmer says, "She's crying, 'It hurts, I'm hungry.' Can you believe it? Only in Haiti would a child cry out that she's hungry during a spinal tap." Later in the book, Kidder writes,

> Haitian doctors, [Farmer] had long ago discovered, learned early to accept all sorts of deficiencies—shortages of medicines, filthy hospitals. Perhaps it is a universal tendency to view the deaths of strangers philosophically. Haitian doctors had better cause for this failing than most others in medicine. Not surprisingly, they tended to shrug when patients died from ailments like measles or tetanus or TB. Farmer had put some of his best efforts into teaching his staff to expect more of themselves. (120)

Elsewhere, writing about Haitian friends of Farmer who had died of preventable diseases, "Each friend had died while in the care of doctors, in the typical, substandard Haitian medical facilities that Farmer had come to loathe" (107). In an episode where a nurse complains that patients do not listen to her instructions, Farmer tells Kidder, "You can't sympathize with the staff too much, or you risk not sympathizing with the patients" (25). These examples suggest that Farmer and presumably other members of PIH, like other foreign individuals and groups working to improve health care in Haiti, have ambivalent and conflicting views of and experiences with Haitian health care workers. On the one hand, the latter are criticized for their complacency and participation in an ineffective system that has failed to provide the most basic health services for the vast majority of Haitians. On the other hand, they are appreciated and valued for the contributions they do make and their unique position to help bring to fruition interventions that international aid groups hope will improve the health of the Haitian poor. This paradox is central to the villain-champion dichotomy I will describe in this chapter.

In writings by and about Farmer, the populations he worked with are characterized primarily by their poverty. This is particularly true in the case of Haitians. Although the majority of Haitians do live in poverty, there are degrees of class stratification within and among the poor. These variations depend on a number of factors including geographic location and proximity infrastructure such as roads and water sources; personal connections and networks within Haiti; and ties to the Haitian diaspora in the United States, Canada, and elsewhere, who send remittances to family members in Haiti and continue to sponsor emigration for their relatives. In addition, analyses of poverty that focus on per capita income or individuals' accumulated wealth ignore the ways that a generalized lack of resources and infrastructure affects not only the poorest of the poor but people in other social categories as well. The physicians, nurses, administrators, health agents, and other hospital employees I studied during my research lived in much better conditions than the patients who typically came to the Justinien (and even better than those populations who did not have the resources to access the hospital). Their lives, however, were also marked by the challenges of living in communities with minimal infrastructure and public resources, and of maintaining a sense of integrity and safety in what the Haitian American author Edwidge Danticat has called the "unraveling" of their country (2008, 115). I would not advance the claim that a surgical nurse and a small-scale market woman experience equivalent levels of suffering due to poverty or structural violence, but it is clear that improving health and economic conditions for Haiti's population depends in no small part on the presence of a professional class in Haiti—health care workers, educators, agronomists, engineers, and others—and that these individuals' experiences and perspectives must be considered in analyses of how health services in Haiti are dispensed.

In pointing out omissions in Farmer's research and publications, my intention is not to discredit him or diminish the quality of the work he produced. Any anthropological account is necessarily incomplete; ethnographers are no longer expected to create accounts detailing all facets of the communities they study. Farmer's decision to focus on the lives and experiences of Haiti's poorest in his research and clinical work is what led him to achieve what few others have. In addition, there is a real risk that resources for PIH/ZL's projects would be diminished or withheld if funders and supporters were to ascertain the tensions, complexities, and failures that are bound to accompany any international aid interventions. In a context of fierce competition between aid organizations for support and funds, there is enormous pressure for those presenting their work to depict it as being the most effective and straightforward. Not doing so could result in being unable to attract new donors or maintain existing ones. This well-founded fear reflects negatively on the will of wealthy governments and societies to commit to acting in lasting solidarity with the world's poor. Farmer would certainly have agreed that the very fact that both his clinical practice and analyses (in particular the premise that all lives should be valued equally) have been considered to be so revolutionary and so desperately needed speaks poorly of existing political, economic, and health care systems.

Medical Heroes as Saintly Figures

In his 2007 book entitled *Giving: How Each of Us Can Change the World*, former US president Bill Clinton wrote: "When I first heard of Paul [Farmer], I asked my daughter, who has a long-standing interest in global health issues, if she knew anything about him. She said, 'Oh Dad, he's a saint. He's our generation's Albert Schweitzer'" (Clinton 2007, 37). Chelsea Clinton's appropriation of Dr. Paul Farmer as her generation's Albert Schweitzer is apt, not only because of specific similarities between the two physicians' lives and work but also because of continuities in how they have been described by observers and commentators. These continuities are particularly striking given the geographic and temporal distances that separate the two men and suggest distinct and recurring patterns in how many North Americans and Europeans conceptualize the work of saintly figures in the field of humanitarian medicine and global health. The combined life spans of these physicians (Schweitzer lived from 1875 to 1965; Farmer was born in 1959), covers a period of enormous changes in how humanitarian medicine is practiced. As extremely visible and influential public figures, both had no small part in shaping these changes.[2] Both have received significant attention from within and beyond the health sector, and both have been (and continue to be) models and inspirational figures for individuals working in the areas of international aid, development, humanitarian intervention, ethics, and global health.

While Farmer and Schweitzer are exceptional as individuals, both in terms of their personal traits and the influence they have had on others, an analysis of these physicians and their work informs our understanding of the roles and relationships of other individuals who emerge as saintly figures in international medical aid. Nearly all the North American NGOs I encountered during my research were founded or are led by a charismatic individual, one who has been particularly successful in garnering resources, recruiting others, and putting medical projects into action. The language of sainthood is frequently used to describe these individuals. While Farmer and Schweitzer are among the most renowned examples, their cases give insight into how certain charismatic individuals working in international health influence others, shape the work of organizations, and become visible as sources of inspiration (and in some instances, controversy). Considering the prominence and epic stature of such figures also draws attention to the relatively low profile of other types of individuals and organizations involved in transnational health interventions, actors who may not be directly involved in the delivery of clinical services, or whose work treating impoverished patients may not involve renunciation, sacrifice, or sainthood in the eyes of outside observers.

While Farmer and Schweitzer as physicians, scholars, and humanitarians may be as different as they are similar, as public figures, the parallels between how they have been described and represented by others are particularly striking. These parallels suggest the existence of enduring and pervasive themes and styles that characterize how certain types of health care workers are represented to and viewed by North American audiences. Other high-profile examples of this figure throughout history include the physicians Norman Bethune (a Canadian who worked in Spain and China in the 1930s and 1940s), and Thomas Dooley (an American who worked in Laos in the 1950s). Most often, these individuals are male physicians, but women and nurses are occasionally represented in a similar light. While physicians in Western societies have held a variety of tangible and symbolic roles over the last two centuries (including healer, entrepreneur, moral authority, genius, social regulator, and others), specific attributes of saintly medical figures include selflessness, altruism, courage, tirelessness, resourcefulness, and compassion. In addition, these individuals have the effect of inspiring others to carry out similar endeavors and initiatives, either through the concrete recruitment of supporters, volunteers, and collaborators, or indirectly through texts and speeches, influential portrayals by others, and reputation more broadly.

In reading about these individuals, several recurring motifs become apparent. The selected examples below are specifically related to Drs. Farmer and Schweitzer but are present in depictions of other medical heroes.

The first of these is the idea that the international medical hero fulfills specific needs beyond those of the population he or she is directly serving as a clinician. Commentators describe a need to have such figures to emulate or even simply to admire. Norman Cousins wrote,

> If Albert Schweitzer is a myth, the myth is more important than the reality. For mankind needs such an image in order to exist. People need to believe that man will sacrifice for man, that he is willing to walk the wide earth in the service of man. Albert Schweitzer is a spiritual immortal. We can be glad that this is so. Each age has need of its saints. A saint becomes a saint when he is claimed by many men as their own, when he awakens in them a desire to know the best that is in them, and the desire to soar morally.... At Lambaréné I learned that a man does not have to be an angel to be a saint. (Cousins 1960, 220)

Echoing this sentiment, C. M. Ballard wrote: "Europeans have needed the reassurance of the old man at Lambaréné." His image "left us with a feeling of pleasure that he was there, in some way representing the things which we would have been doing if other responsibilities had not forbidden it" (1965, 225). Similarly, on a website featuring the work of Paul Farmer, one reads, "Society needs heroes to rejuvenate, re-energize and renew itself with visions of the possible. That's what heroes do" (www.myhero.com). In this way, the saintly doctors' patients are not the only ones to benefit from their work; anyone who comes in contact with them (directly or indirectly) and is inspired to emulate them benefits from an opportunity for self-improvement.

A second motif is that of renunciation and self-sacrifice, which appear commonly in writings about both Farmer and Schweitzer. Before beginning their work abroad, both lived in relatively privileged conditions, and benefited from affiliations with powerful institutions. Commentators assume and explicitly state that they could have stayed in their native environments and enjoyed the material comforts available to them. Authors highlight that both had accomplished a great deal at an unusually young age, and therefore could have enjoyed rewarding careers and a high standard of living in their respective places of origin. Writers who visited Lambaréné and Cange often described in detail the simple and rudimentary living situations that these doctors chose over upper-class dwellings in Europe and the United States (Schweitzer's piano was often mentioned as a quaint anomaly in his otherwise Spartan residence).

About Farmer, Kidder writes: "Obviously, a young man with his advantages could have been doing good works as a doctor while commuting between Boston and a pleasant suburb—not between a room in what I imagined must be a grubby church rectory and the wasteland of central Haiti. The way he talked, it seemed he actually enjoyed living among Haitian peasant farmers" (Kidder 2003, 7). The decision to pursue medical projects in impoverished settings when doing so is neither financially lucrative nor physically comfortable is described by authors and observers as one that, for these men, was not inevitable but reflected a conscious choice. A paradox ensues where the hero becomes successful and influential ostensibly by rejecting more conventional means of becoming successful and influential. A central early narrative about Farmer and the cofounders of Partners in Health is that they were underdogs in the world of international health: as medical students and young volunteers founding a small organization. Today PIH and its sister organizations represent a significant source of health care in the countries where they operate, having received over 200 million USD in revenue in 2020. While this amount is dwarfed by the sums earned by corporations or spent on national militaries, it is fair to say that Farmer was and PIH continues to be a major player in the field of global health.

A third prominent theme in depictions of international medical heroes is a confrontation with danger in some form. In the cases of Farmer and Schweitzer, Africa and Haiti represent for many observers a confrontation with poverty, an unfamiliar and uncomfortable climate, a lack of material comforts, risks of political and social instability, and contact with African and Afro-Caribbean populations infamous for their alleged "savagery," lack of civilization, and use of malicious magic. The confrontation with danger is heightened in descriptions of Farmer and Schweitzer by accentuating certain conditions and personal characteristics: their youth, their lack of prior experience in such impoverished settings, and their relative isolation from other foreigners during their early encounters. With patience, courage, and charisma, the international medical hero is able to resolve difficult situations, build relationships with locals for collaboration, and eventually gain a certain amount of influence in a harsh and potentially hostile environment.

Although Schweitzer and Farmer are two of the most prominent examples of medical heroes as saintly figures, the archetype is also applicable to individuals working on a much smaller scale and with much less visibility. In Haiti as in other contexts, these individuals often tend to be male physicians, whose work is usually supported by medical and nonmedical group members whose professional status, age, and experience in Haiti were frequently less than that of the hero. (I did meet several women who were international medical heroes in Haiti, and, with increasing rates of women in the medical profession, it seems likely that this figure will become less exclusively male with time.) Nearly all the individuals occupying organizations' leadership roles, however, were physicians. While North American NGOs working on issues related to education, food, child welfare, and evangelization were often spearheaded by nonprofessionals, the degree of hierarchy and specialization in medicine made it difficult for someone other than a high-status clinician to assume a leadership role in medical interventions. Heroic figures were not a prominent feature in all the groups and agencies I studied; interventions by governmental and large multinational agencies were more often implemented by individuals in subordinate and heavily bureaucratized positions than by charismatic leaders. In smaller, nongovernmental groups, however, members of the organizations were nearly always able to identify a "driving force" for their group—a founder, director, or volunteer whose energy and initiative were essential to the functioning of the organization and to the implementation of interventions.

The centrality of a single individual in the functioning and success of international medical aid organizations was described both positively and negatively by the group members I interviewed. For the most part, the leaders' roles and relationships with other members resulted from individuals' personal traits and characteristics—NGOs' fairly flexible structures and governance allowed individuals to negotiate a position in the group that corresponded to their interests, availabilities, and personalities. Many individuals told me that they preferred to take what they called "supporting roles," and let someone else lead and make decisions. Generally, the leaders were appreciated by their groups' members, who looked up to them and were grateful for their work and leadership, although some members expressed concern about their group's future in the case of the leader's inability to carry out his or her functions. In the case of aging individuals, many aid workers and volunteers expressed concern about the future of their groups and initiatives after the retirement or death of their charismatic leaders.

Although most of the groups I observed maintained relatively harmonious organizational relationships, some evidence of conflicts related to centralized leadership emerged. Prior to my research, two major actors in a small medical NGO had had a major conflict over the group's leadership and priorities, with one nurse who ultimately left the organization accusing the other leader of "killing my baby" (in other words, making significant changes to the group's structure and functioning). Conflicts among international members of aid groups most frequently revolved around prioritization of activities, management of resources, and differences in personality and perspectives. It is not uncommon to find organizations in Haiti (and elsewhere) that began as offshoots or splinter movements of previously existing groups, either in the context of intense conflicts or more subtle divergences in projects and priorities.

In sum, charismatic, saintly leaders are both visible as internationally prominent figures (such as Schweitzer and Farmer) and on a smaller scale, in the everyday workings of transnational medical aid and humanitarian organizations. The language of sainthood suggests a number of features associated with representations of these individuals: extraordinary powers and talents to accomplish tasks that seem insurmountable by ordinary people; an exceptional level of commitment or devotion to the cause they have chosen; and, finally, a degree of distinction or apartness, not only from their communities of origin but also from the populations in which they intervene. To achieve saintly status in working with impoverished Haitians, one can neither be impoverished nor Haitian. Saintly status is premised on renunciation (and therefore having a position to renounce). It is also dependent on a level of arbitrariness in the choice of population one is aiding. Helping one's own national group, for example, carries with it the connotation of patriotism and self-interest, which taint the motivations to do "pure" good. Charismatic individuals working in Haiti who identify as Haitian are preemptively excluded from the category of saint and are much more likely to be portrayed as either villains or champions.

Villains

Perhaps because attributing the label of villain to a specific individual would be considered an act of hostility, or simply because they are reviled figures, one hears much less about villains than saints in the official discourse and representations of aid programs. Villains in the context of humanitarian encounters can have several manifestations. One is that of the undeserving recipient, an individual whose needs are not as pressing or serious as another person's, and who nonetheless receives aid. Examples could include a person who receives food aid despite having enough to eat, or someone who accepts or obtains a donation of medication despite not having the treatment's targeted ailment. In such cases, one can imagine undeserving recipients justifying accumulating excess resources in case of future needs, or in order to exchange or redistribute them later. The latter could be a morally acceptable action since a person in need would ultimately receive the resource, but the practice of recipients reselling donated items for monetary gain is often named as a symptom of aid gone wrong, either because the aid did not correspond to the population's needs, or because the population receiving aid is not in need.

While benefiting from humanitarian resources in and of itself is not necessarily immoral, the stakes change significantly when one is surrounded by others who are in real need. While definitions of stealing and theft vary greatly, taking possessions or resources from others is condemned in a wide range of legal and moral systems. Stealing from the rich to give to the poor is sometimes presented as a noble act, however, taking from those who are needier than oneself is rarely considered an acceptable action. A nurse who would use funds from a community nutrition program to pay for her own children's school fees, a hospital administrator who sells donated medicines that were intended for free distribution, a doctor who sees patients for high fees during hours when she is paid by an NGO to see destitute patients free of charge: these are all examples of behaviors that both Haitians and foreigners find to be morally reprehensible. The higher the status of the person stealing or diverting the resources, the more condemnable the act. In other words, if a community health worker were to pilfer resources that were intended for distribution, such behavior might be considered "understandable" by donors, who would recognize that the worker, whose remuneration is quite low, may be living in conditions similar to those of the impoverished individuals for whom the goods were donated. In the case of a physician who would commit a similar act, his or her status, revenue (real or perceived), and relative distance from the population of recipients would make this act more immoral than if it had been committed by someone with less means.

In the context of international aid, therefore, the archetypal villain is marked by both proximity and distance from the victim. One on level, the villain must be close enough to the victims to have witnessed the latter's poverty and suffering and to have an understanding of the consequences of one's evil actions. On another level, a villain cannot be too close to victims in economic status or social conditions, as his or her self-serving actions would then become based on desperation and need. In Haiti, as in other impoverished settings, those in the category of "local elites"—whether they be health professionals, government officials, merchants and businesspeople, clergy, or other categories—are frequently scrutinized by foreigners for their moral valence and the perception that their wealth, power, and success are particularly condemnable if they exist in geographic proximity to poverty.

The fact that existing as a person with resources in the context of extreme poverty can make one subject to condemnation by others is illustrated by the following banal encounter. One Sunday afternoon during my first summer in a Haitian village, I came across an adolescent boy whose leg had been badly burned when he walked into a street vendor's pot of hot cooking oil. A large patch of infected skin on his leg was black and charred. I asked him why he had not been to the small local hospital, and he said that he did not have the money to pay the consultation fee. Horrified by the severity of his wound and infuriated by the situation, I told him that I would go with him to the hospital and make sure he got care. When we arrived at the hospital, the building was empty, except for a lone security guard. I asked him if he could go alert the hospital's only physician, who lived on the hospital grounds. I walked with the guard toward the physician's room and overheard a sentence of their brief exchange. "Tell him I'm asleep!" the physician told the guard. I remember my feeling of righteous indignation at that moment and the sense of injustice that came from the realization that a medical doctor would deny care to someone in need. It was very clear in my mind who was the villain and who was the victim, and whose side I was on. Only later did I consider that, as the only physician for a population of over eighty thousand, and being elderly and in poor health himself, this physician may have been justified in setting limits on his availability to provide care for others. After his death several years later, he was remembered in the community not as the most generous or caring doctor but was appreciated simply because he stayed in the area when he could have emigrated to a city or abroad. In this case, the boy recovered from his injuries, but others were not so lucky.

When an individual is permanently disabled by or dies because of a lack of care, how is blame attributed? A good Samaritan is clearly good because of her or his intervention, but what of those who could conceivably help but do not? As noted by William Olsen and Thomas Csordas in their 2019 edited volume, anthropologists have been reticent to directly address the question of evil, in part because of the term's roots in European moral traditions. A growing number of anthropologists have explored the concept of corruption and its related practices (Smith 2008; Muir and Gupta 2018), however medical anthropologists and anthropologists of global health have tended to identify depersonalized forces such as political economy of health or structural violence in creating and exacerbating health inequalities.

It is important to note that both the saint and villain categories are contingent on others' appraisals. Individuals who proclaim their own sainthood threaten to lose their status, as humility, modesty, and self-effacement are valued (particularly in the Judeo-Christian tradition) over pride, boasting, and self-promotion. Figures designated as saints by others can promote their activities, make visible the results of their work, and draw attention to partners and beneficiaries, however, explicit proclamations of one's own moral rectitude risks being interpreted as an attempt to gain personal power and influence, and can even draw suspicious attention to what one might be hiding or trying to distract from. Conversely, no one would have an interest in promoting one's own villainous behavior in the context of humanitarian aid, as doing so could lead to moral condemnation by others, legal sanctions, or even violence. In considering who has saint or villain status, it is essential to keep in mind who is making these characterizations, and what criteria are used to make these designations. During my fieldwork in Haiti, I heard both foreigners and Haitians (particularly of the middle and lower classes) making accusations against wealthy Haitians, naming the latter's large homes, expensive cars, travels abroad, and lavish lifestyles as signs that they had taken more than their fair share of resources or failed in their duty to redistribute them and live modest lifestyles that would reduce the gaps between them and their impoverished compatriots. The irony, of course, is that many of the foreigners I met who traveled to Haiti to volunteer or to work in the health and development sectors there lived fairly privileged lifestyles in their home countries, and (particularly in Port-au-Prince) earned high salaries and lived in opulent conditions themselves. However, the characterization of individuals from wealthy countries—particularly white persons—who travel to Haiti to work in the health sector is of self-sacrifice and devotion to others, regardless of the conditions they live in or the work they accomplish.

The "People of Color" and the "Little Whites"

The condemnation of elites in Haiti can be considered in historical context. While over two hundred years have elapsed since Haiti gained its independence from France, and although color and class formations in the Caribbean are undergoing continuous changes, the systems and hierarchies established during the colonial period cast long shadows that have profoundly shaped Haitian society and the country's relations with other nations (Trouillot 1990). In Saint-Domingue, the French colony that would eventually become the Republic of Haiti, economy and society were organized around a violent system of agricultural plantations and resource extraction. Enslaved Africans and their descendants toiled in abominable conditions on French-owned plantations. While many of the plantations belonged to absentee owners who never left Europe, others were owned or administered by whites who had migrated or were born in the colonies of settler parents. Historians present a dichotomy between the *grands blancs* (which included landowners, aristocrats, powerful businessmen, and the clergy) and *petits blancs*, poorer individuals who came to Saint-Domingue as indentured servants, manual laborers, artisans, sailors, petty tradesmen, and fortune seekers. Over time, a population of mixed-race individuals emerged—initially as the children of violent unions between European men and enslaved African women—whose identities were determined according to a complex system of racial classification (Moreau de Saint-Méry [1789] 1958). These individuals, often referred to with the terms *mulâtres* (mulattoes) or *gens de couleur* (people of color) occupied a wide range of positions in colonial Saint-Domingue. While some were born into slavery and would remain so for their entire lives, others were recognized by their fathers, sent to Europe for their formal education, and would eventually occupy high positions in the colonial system, owning their own slaves and plantations.

While the most visible and dramatic narratives of Saint-Domingue's colonial history and the Haitian Revolution understandably focus on oppression by the French and the successful revolt against them by enslaved Africans and their descendants, this dichotomy hides the tensions between other categories of individuals in the same way that models of humanitarianism which focus only on wealthy donors and impoverished recipients leave out crucial components of aid processes. In this context, it is important to note that some of the most violent conflicts in colonial Saint-Domingue took place between *gens de couleur* and *petits blancs*; in other words, the elite of a racially subaltern population and the lowest classes of a racially dominant group (L. Dubois 2004, 70, 84–88). This makes sense, when one considers that the highest and lowest members of any hierarchy are rarely in direct contact or confrontation. When would the wealthiest absentee plantation owners come into contact with their human property, the enslaved men and women on Saint-Domingue's sugar plantations? Frictions were much more likely to erupt between the lighter-skinned and wealthy mulattoes who "dared" to access power in a system that questioned their very humanity, and those poor whites who possessed none of the material means or social status that corresponded to the place they felt they should be afforded at the top of the colonial racial hierarchy.

Central conflicts during the colonial period revolved around whites restricting the access of nonwhites to certain echelons of political and economic power, judgments made on the moral and intellectual capacities of different groups based on racialized classifications, and the relations whites and nonwhite elites would have with those who were enslaved. In the early nineteenth century, under the looming threat of American influence and invasion, Haitian intellectuals would justify the discrepancy between their francophilia and the nation's colonial past by arguing that the *colons* in Saint-Domingue represented the dregs of French society (Hoffman 1984). This position allowed members of Haiti's elite to condemn certain Europeans' actions and character while maintaining an admiration for specific dimensions of European culture and thought. The American marine occupation of Haiti, which lasted from 1915 to 1934, deepened the mutual mistrust by elite Haitians and white foreigners. Suzy Castor (1988) argues that the Haitian elite, despite its prejudice against the country's Black majority, did not consider themselves inferior to their white American occupants, and were particularly angered by the practices of racial segregation installed by foreigners in their country (96–97). The historian Brenda Gayle Plummer describes what she calls the

"Anglo-American disdain for mulattoes," which was furthered by the "belief that such persons, as links between the races, endangered the established order in what should be a rigidly color-defined world. . . . Mulattoes thus constituted a multiple challenge, which could only be met by impugning their personal worth. The conspicuous failures of the Haitian bourgeoisie as a leadership class greatly assisted with this denial, but the terms of rejection had more to do with what 'Negroes' were supposed to be. . . . Their critics mourned a lost world where blacks knew their place and did not boast frock coats and Sorbonne doctorates" (1992, 128–29).

The themes of these conflicts are echoed in the relationships between higher-status Haitians and foreigners today, although comparisons and juxtapositions should not be taken as equivalencies. Historical tensions between populations in colonial Saint-Domingue or early twentieth-century US-occupied Haiti do not map neatly onto contemporary frictions between Haitian health professionals and foreigners. Thinking about international interventions in historical context, however, raises an important question: What is at stake in the moral assessments made about wealthy and powerful individuals in poor countries by foreigners who claim to be intervening in the interests of the poorest citizens of those countries?

The expression "Morally Repugnant Elites" or "Most Repugnant Elites" attests to the judgment cast on Haiti's elite by English-speaking foreigners. I was unable to determine the specific origin of the expression, but it does not seem to have a commonly used French equivalent; it may have been coined by American diplomats, journalists, or aid workers. (In French-language texts, writers often specify that *l'élite la plus répugnante* is a translation of the English term.) Haitian elites are aware of this moniker, and as one of them stated, "We are not the most repugnant elite, we are equally repugnant!" (Fatton 2002, xii). A 1994 *New York Times* article cited another individual who attempted to situate his social class vis-à-vis the citizens of other countries. "I made a lot of money in this country," said Ronald A. Georges, aged thirty-seven, a wholesaler of Lebanese descent who was born and reared in Haiti. "I have a nice house. I didn't steal. I didn't cheat. People in America have nice houses. But they talk about us as M.R.E.'s: the morally repugnant elite. I'm sick and tired of being called an M.R.E. I'm not saying we are Boy Scouts. But we made money by working" (Manegold 1994). (It should be noted that Ronald Georges was found guilty of financial crimes and sentenced to a year in prison in 2007.)

It is undeniable that some members of powerful families in Haiti have committed reprehensible acts throughout the country's history: they have supported dictatorships and violent military bodies, they have acted in ways that have perpetuated racist hierarchies and the exclusion of the majority of Haiti's population from participation in civic and political life, and they have contributed to the suffering and misery of millions of their fellow citizens. These are not conspiratorial or fanciful claims; they are based on empirical research and evidence, sometimes collected and presented by scholars and activists who grew up as members of the very social class they condemn. Other members of these same families have contributed significantly to improving the lives of impoverished Haitians: supporting progressive causes, devoting their careers to furthering social justice. These choices often come at a price. Estelle told me that, while her siblings were supportive and admiring of her involvement in providing health services in rural Haiti, members of her extended family cut off ties with her because they felt that, as she put it, "It's not our place to do that." Others have paid with their lives: the businessman Antoine Izméry, one of Haiti's wealthiest businessmen and an opponent of the 1991–94 military coup regime, was assassinated in 1993. There is no doubt that the system that creates such extreme inequalities in Haiti and around the world is violent and unjust; how specific individuals navigate their place in these inequalities is a much more complicated matter.

It is important to note that, while foreign aid workers may classify wealthier Haitians as villains because of their relationship to poverty and misery, which is at once close and distant, middle- and upper-class Haitians, conversely, will cast judgments on the foreigners who come to Haiti with the stated purpose of encountering or alleviating this same poverty and misery. The middle- and upper-class Haitians I encountered accused foreigners of ignorance of Haiti's history and social context, of racism disguised as benevolence, and of the same greed and exploitative tendencies that they themselves were accused of. They often found North Americans in particular to be crass and unsophisticated, eager to take action and direct others but lacking in awareness of the social codes and the intricacies of relationships and networks that govern interactions in the Haitian context. From this perspective, it is the foreigners who are the villains, although—perhaps because of my own identity as a foreigner—my Haitian interlocutors were adamant in making a distinction between good and bad foreigners.

The villain category is not the only one available to Haitian professionals. As noted earlier, young physicians in Haiti today are generally not from the country's elite class, but rather from a middle class that relies heavily on ties to the diaspora for financial support. Their proximity to poorer members of the population and their ability to engage with transnational organizations as local professionals renders them eligible to be classified in a third category: champions.

Champions

In the organizations I studied, Haitians and members of the Haitian diaspora occasionally acted as a group's central, charismatic, and heroic figure, particularly for organizations that were smaller, less visible, and consisted mostly of Haitian and diaspora Haitian members. In the case of larger and more prominent organizations, they tended to occupy secondary and subordinate roles. Examples include the Haitian American physician who directed a university-based initiative to provide HIV+ positive patients with medical services, including antiretroviral medications; the community health agent who emerged as a local authority figure and spokeswoman, looking after neighborhood children and organizing her area's residents to pressure municipal authorities into channeling resources to their neighborhood's minimal infrastructure; the Haitian medical resident whose charismatic personality, intelligence, and dedication made her an obvious choice for an American organization seeking out a local partner for research and intervention; and the Cuban-trained Haitian physician who was appointed medical director of a rural hospital that operates out of a partnership between a US-based NGO and the Haitian Ministry of Health.

Some of the characteristics of saintly international aid workers also apply to Haitian clinicians who emerge as charismatic figures, with extraordinary intellectual and clinical talents, strong interpersonal skills, and a proven commitment to the health of the poor. There were also some important differences. The aspect of renunciation central to achieving a saintly status is particularly complicated in Haiti, where only a small segment of the population would be able to renounce material gain, resources, and opportunities commensurate with the renunciation of their international colleagues. Most Haitians do not have lucrative jobs or a secure, comfortable lifestyle to renounce in the first place. Even Haitian medical professionals, whose living conditions and future prospects are inarguably better than most of their compatriots, struggle with debt, insecurity, and the pressures and demands related to supporting their families and kin networks. In a context where obligations and loyalty toward *moun pa* (one's people) are a defining feature of one's identity and life choices, and where failure to maintain networks through the redistribution of capital, resources, and services can have devastating consequences, it is particularly difficult for Haitian health workers to renounce professional and economic advancement. Choosing not to support one's own, whether defined in kin, community, or national terms, is considered to be particularly egregious moral failing in Haiti.

Even more striking is the contrast between international medical aid workers' and Haitian health professionals' prospects in terms of national destinies. Turmoil in Haiti for a foreign clinician can be mitigated by a return to one's home country and a shift toward prior or alternate occupations. Haitian clinicians, however, particularly those lacking the status and documentation needed to travel or work abroad, are much more vulnerable to the negative outcomes of instability and what many describe as Haiti's dismal future prospects. Even having renounced professional or personal objectives, the international medical worker or volunteer can feasibly choose to return to a secure lifestyle in his or her country of origin; this scenario is not as possible for clinicians from Haiti or other impoverished settings.

Nevertheless, Haitian clinicians do, of course, make a wide range of renunciations, and some of these are noticed and appreciated by outside observers. In the case of health workers who have emigrated and return to Haiti either permanently or periodically to be involved in aid, both Haitians and non-Haitians often remark that the person in question was not contractually obligated to return to their home country, and that many members of the diaspora are minimally or not at all involved in efforts to improve their home country. Another group includes health workers who had the possibility of emigrating but chose not to, or those who make professional choices to serve needy segments of Haiti's population instead of or in addition to providing better remunerated care to wealthier patients. These individuals are described by observers as *dedicated* or *devoted*, terms that echo the language of sainthood when applied to certain foreigners intervening in Haiti.

While renunciation is a component of medical heroism that is often applied by observers to the experiences of Haitian clinicians (albeit it in modified form), confrontation with danger is rarely mentioned in representations of the latter's work, particularly in comparison with depictions of foreign aid workers. This may stem from the fact that, for most foreigners, their very presence in Haiti as non-Haitians is considered to be the riskiest aspect of their work. This loses its relevance when discussing Haitian and diaspora health workers, who are already in the country or familiar with it from living there previously. The purported "danger" foreigners experience in Haiti is often expressed in terms of class and race—an immersion among poor people of African ancestry—a situation that many international aid workers assume is a nonissue for Haitian health workers. In talking with Haitian clinicians, however, I found that many of them found experiences such as working in rural areas or parts of the country they were unfamiliar with to be extremely disconcerting, especially at first. While most eventually adapted to being outside an urban area and separated from their families, nearly all found these experiences trying on a number of levels, including isolation, adaptation to new surroundings and challenging living conditions, and a lack of basic infrastructure in their living and working environments. In addition, health workers and other professionals felt extremely vulnerable and targeted by the waves of kidnappings that began in 2005 and continue to target not only wealthier Haitians but middle-class and poorer individuals as well. Medical professionals have been targeted in more recent kidnappings in 2020 and 2021, during periods of heightened insecurity and instability. Many foreigners

I met in Haiti were not aware of the degree of fear these kidnappings had pro-voked among Haitian health professionals or the extent to which the latter had been affected by them. Overall, they considered their own travel to and activities in Haiti to be a dramatic confrontation with various forms of danger, whereas Haitian professionals' presence in the country was generally considered more matter-of-fact and mundane.

Rather than saints, therefore, Haitian health professionals are often relegated to a secondary archetypal category, that of the *champion*. The term has been used in an increasing number of areas; from its original meaning referring to a fighter or combatant, it is now mostly associated with athletic performance, or with aspirations of excellence among students and young people, at least in its North American usage. It was during my research at a US medical school's global health training program that I became aware of the use of this term in the global health field. While attending global health courses and conferences, it was common for instructors and panelists to end their presentation with a "Lessons Learned" Pow-erPoint slide that gave aspiring global health students and practitioners advice and warnings deemed useful in planning global health interventions. One of the "Lessons Learned" that appeared repeatedly in these presentations was to "find local champions" for their global health projects. The "local champions" were individuals based in the countries or communities where the intervention would be taking place. While the speakers did not always make explicit what qualities characterized these local champions, their presence was essential for ensuring the success of the project. They could act as translators and cultural brokers, navigat-ing between students and clinicians from the global North and the population in the global South who would presumably function in unintelligible languages and unfamiliar social codes. Local champions could also facilitate bureaucracies and logistics, drawing on their knowledge of formal and informal structures for get-ting things done. Finally, these individuals could become the spokespeople and promoters for global health initiatives, which would come to be perceived as ini-tiatives that were at least partly local, as opposed to being imposed from abroad.

I suspect that one of the reasons why the idea of the local champion is so popular in health care is that so many medical aid and global health projects *do* rely on the participation and contribution of actors in the sites of intervention, and that these individuals *do* stand out for their charisma, abilities in communi-cation, resourcefulness, and personality. In every medical aid project I encoun-tered in Haiti, a champion figure was immediately identifiable. Sometimes these individuals held relatively prominent and powerful roles in the organization; at other times, their status was much closer to that of a service worker or domes-tic servant. Their roles and responsibilities included picking up visiting medi-cal teams at the airport; securing lodging and arranging for meals; coordinating communications with other Haiti-based staff; facilitating contacts in hospitals and clinics; setting up mobile and temporary clinics in schools and churches; and working alongside foreigners as clinicians, translators, and fixers. When the foreign teams were absent, champions contributed to projects by recruiting patients in need of specialized care. Much of the champions' work involved facilitating the functioning of international project staff and volunteers in the context of limited infrastructure, and smoothing over relationships between expatriates and key individuals and institutions in Haiti: patients, government authorities, and Haitian employees of other establishments and organizations. Champions are central to establishing and maintaining partnerships, one of the most commonly used terms to describe relationships between northern and southern institutions and governments in the context of global health. Johanna Crane (2013, 161–71) has detailed the ambiguities surrounding the term *partnership* in this realm, specifically the diversity of configurations and relationships it can refer to and the inequalities it can reinforce in postcolonial settings.

Recognizing champions' subordinate position is not to say that they do not receive recognition for their efforts. In fact, they are increasingly featured in promotion campaigns, newsletters, fundraising appeals, and annual reports, so much that portrayals of champions have developed a predictable, almost scripted form. When a foreign NGO publishes an interview with a Haitian nurse or health agent, they do so in a fairly predictable way: the champion is asked about his or her biography (if it involves a humble or modest background, this is often highlighted); and they often present the community where they work, stressing the challenges and difficulties they and their patients might face. The interview or feature often closes with the champion describing the favorite part of their job, the impact the organization they work with has made, or their hopes for the future.

The distinction between a saint and a champion is not absolute, and, in many cases, a person could be classified as either. But making a distinction between the two categories allows for certain patterns to emerge. Notably, we can see how and why certain people emerge as visible and influential actors in the context of humanitarianism and aid, and why others work in relative obscurity. In relation to the populations they are helping, saints have a certain removed, otherworldly quality. Their distinction is marked by a number of attributes: in Haiti, saints tend to be white and from wealthier countries. Their contact with countries like Haiti emerged through chance encounters. Champions, on the other hand, are considered in some way to be *of* the group they are helping. They may have accrued distance through social mobility or migration, but in terms of their origins, champions in Haiti are Haitian; their choice to intervene in Haiti is not circumstantial, but rather tied to their identity as Haitians or members of the Haitian diaspora. Whereas saints may have easier access to international resources, champions must work harder to stand out and be noticed. In addition, champions regularly run the risk of losing their status and being reclassified as villains, particularly if they behave in ways that are not in accordance with their employer's objectives and values.

Moral Outsourcing and the White Savior Industrial Complex

The archetypical figures I have described are not restricted to humanitarian aid or global health. Though their particular characteristics vary across social and cultural contexts, heroic and antiheroic figures help structure narratives, offer examples of moral and immoral conduct, and give meaning to human experience. In offering a critical analysis of archetypical figures in humanitarianism and global health, I am not suggesting that they do not serve important and necessary purposes: saints, villains, and champions inspire, challenge, and caution those around them in ways that can lead to improved interventions and great equity. However, I am concerned by the prominence of these figures in global health and the attention that is given to individuals' traits at the expense of broader structures and patterns—either those that worsen health conditions (extractive capitalism, systemic racism, gender inequalities) or those that work to improve them (political resistance movements, education programs, health systems reforms). By imagining global health as resting on the efforts of extraordinary singular individuals, reducing health inequalities takes on the proportion of colossal tasks, tasks that cannot be accomplished by ordinary people, collective action, or institutions and structures. This perception, that one must be a physician (or a genius, or a millionaire, or a professor, or a member of an elite group) to generate changes or combat injustice can lead to a sort of moral outsourcing: a tendency to consider the reduction of health and other inequities as the purview of a select group of individuals rather than a shared civic and human responsibility.

In addition to the passivity that comes with moral outsourcing, one can also examine the negative consequences of holding up individuals as saints when we consider the aspirations and trajectories of young people interested in participating in positive social change. An incessant emphasis on global health leaders and heroes conveys not only the idea that charismatic, individual actions are the best models for creating social change but also that failures or enduring problems are the results of individual failures. Current models of humanitarian and global health interventions implicitly send the message that certain individuals are to be admired and emulated, while others (namely, corrupt elites or indifferent bureaucrats) must be tolerated, avoided, or actively combated. Holding up extraordinary figures as exemplars also sends the message that everyday actions and ordinary individuals cannot lead to social change. In the wave of interest and enthusiasm for global health that has swept across North American universities in the last two decades, we have not considered what will happen to those students who do not rise to prominence, who do not graduate at the top of their class or pursue MD-PhD degrees. Will it lead to a number of "global-health dropouts" for whom the reductive model of extreme performance and renunciation were never an option?

While local actors' critiques of conventional aid models have circulated in communities for decades, public critiques of aid and, in particular, of the saint archetype have become increasingly visible in recent years, facilitated by the rapid communications afforded by internet-based social media. In 2012, in response to the viral documentary film *Kony 2012*, the Nigerian American author Teju Cole wrote a series of tweets and a follow-up article in the *Atlantic* about what he called the "white savior industrial complex." While Cole's arguments mostly refer to Africa, their relevance for the Haitian context is obvious:

> One song we hear too often is the one in which Africa serves as a backdrop for white fantasies of conquest and heroism. From the colonial project to *Out of Africa* to *The Constant Gardener* and *Kony 2012*, Africa has provided a space onto which white egos can conveniently be projected. It is a liberated space in which the usual rules do not apply: a nobody from America or Europe can go to Africa and become a godlike savior or, at the very least, have his or her emotional needs satisfied. Many have done it under the banner of "making a difference." To state this obvious and well-attested truth does not make me a racist or a Mau. It does give me away as an "educated middle-class African," and I plead guilty as charged. (Cole 2012)

Cole quotes the *New York Times* journalist Nicholas Kristof's remarks to the former's original critical tweets, which explicitly named Kristof as representing the white savior industrial complex:

> There has been a real discomfort and backlash among middle-class educated Africans, Ugandans in particular in this case, but people more broadly, about having Africa as they see it defined by a warlord who does particularly brutal things, and about the perception that Americans are going to ride in on a white horse and resolve it. To me though, it seems even more uncomfortable to think that we as white Americans

> should not intervene in a humanitarian disaster because the victims are
> of a different skin color. (Kristof, quoted in Cole 2012)

The oppositions that are set up in this exchange illustrate the ways that tensions in international interventions and aid are expressed through morally laden archetypes, in this case "middle-class educated Africans," who, while not explicitly villainized by Kristof, are implicitly critiqued for not recognizing the more "uncomfortable" prospect than skewed definitions or perceptions: a potential *lack* of intervention by white Americans.

It is difficult to develop critical perspectives on international medical interventions knowing that so many people in Haiti and elsewhere are lacking in basic biomedical resources. There are tremendous pressures and reasons simply to augment care, services, materials, and personnel, particularly when one has seen the crowded waiting rooms and poorly stocked pharmacies of Haitian dispensaries, clinics, and hospitals. Yet if the response to the 2010 earthquake and cholera epidemic has taught us anything, it is that the amount of aid pledged—whether in financial, material, or human resources—cannot be considered separately from the ways it is disbursed, the channels through which it travels, and the health systems it strengthens, bypasses, or undermines. The importance of health systems was further highlighted during the 2013–16 West African Ebola outbreak, when insufficient health structures and human resources made every dimension of the epidemic more challenging—prevention of new cases, diagnosis, and treatment—despite significant levels of international intervention and aid. The same realization has become apparent in ways that we are only beginning to grasp during the COVID-19 pandemic. It remains to be seen whether the tenacious dichotomies of saints and victims will give way to a conception of global health that takes seriously the work and priorities of local health professionals, not just as potential champions or victims, but as legitimate and agentive actors in developing integrated health systems to care for their populations.

CONCLUSION

When I finished the initial fieldwork research for this study in the spring of 2009, I had no way of knowing that geological forces would transform the subject of my work—medical aid to Haiti—from a relatively obscure topic to one that would receive unprecedented attention in the international media. On January 12, 2010, a catastrophic earthquake measuring 7.0 on the Richter scale struck southern Haiti, devastating Port-au-Prince and its surrounding areas. Estimates for casualties ranged from between 50,000 and 300,000, although a lack of reliable census data, the inability to retrieve many of the victims' bodies, and the internment of thousands of corpses in mass graves make the exact number impossible to calculate (OCHA 2011). The loss of infrastructure was also devastating: twenty-eight out of twenty-nine government ministry buildings collapsed during the quake and its aftershocks (MacFarquhar 2010), and countless homes, workplaces, schools, and churches were reduced to rubble, which, for years after the quake, continued to impede the rebuilding process and even the most basic flows of circulation and traffic.

In the days that followed the quake, the medical response from abroad was swift and spectacular. Working under the auspices of governmental and nongovernmental agencies, disaster, rescue, and emergency medical teams freed Haitians from under trapped buildings, set up temporary hospitals in tents and hangars, and worked to save earthquake victims from death by blood loss, infections, and shock. With hundreds of thousands of people injured, the need for medical care far outweighed available medical resources; it is impossible to know how many people died from lack of basic care. The most common injuries were caused by falling walls and collapsing buildings—victims were treated for blunt trauma and crushed limbs. A relief worker described many of the wounds as "tiger slashes"—these were usually vertical gouges from falling cinder blocks. In the weeks and months that followed, after the patients with traumatic injuries had either been treated or died from their injuries, the population's medical needs returned to their tragic prequake banality: waterborne infections (exacerbated by water scarcity in crowded tent camps), complications related to pregnancy and childbirth, and the ongoing ravages of malnutrition and unsafe living conditions.

I returned to Haiti shortly after the earthquake, initially in Cap-Haïtien and eventually translating for American relief workers at a field hospital set up on the grounds of the Port-au-Prince airport. Cap-Haïtien, like most of the country, had not sustained any direct structural damage from the earthquake, but the population was still reeling from the shock of losing relatives, of the economic perturbations the quake engendered, and the ramifications the catastrophe had for the country's political and economic life. Medical activities in the north were seriously affected. Many of the earthquake victims made their way to their regions of origin with the help of family members and friends, and before long, NGOs were involved in the transportation of people needing medical care to hospitals in the area. As in other Haitian cities, municipal officials in Cap-Haïtien arranged for the transport of people from the area who had migrated to the capital, including injured people requiring medical care. The Hôpital Sacré-Coeur in nearby Milot received hundreds of patients, drawing on their capacity to integrate foreign medical teams in their work and to receive donated supplies from foreign donors. That hospital's administration and board set up tents on the hospital's property to expand their capacity from seventy-five inpatients to nearly four hundred, and US Coast Guard helicopters airlifted injured patients from Port-au-Prince to a makeshift launchpad near the hospital.

At the Justinien, the influx of patients was much less dramatic. The hospital received approximately sixty victims in the days that followed the quake, and the hospital's staff expressed their frustration at the administration's incapacity to respond effectively to the situation. A few days after the earthquake, the hospital's administration became so overwhelmed with offers of aid by foreign agencies, groups, and individuals that they asked Konbit Sante to become the official contact point and liaison with the hospital's international's partners. This act testifies not only to the number of actors involved and the complexity of the situation (one that would compel the hospital's administration to relinquish its strategic position as hub in dealing with international partners) but also to the administrators' appreciation of Konbit Sante, to the extent that they would entrust the American group with a position that required so much careful strategizing and could potentially confer so much power and privileged access to resources and relationships.

Rather than fundamentally alter the processes I have described in this book, the earthquake and the international medical responses to it amplified many of the tendencies and phenomena I observed during my fieldwork. For example, as material donations represented both a source of tangible benefits and sources of conflict before 2010, they continued to do so in the weeks and months after the quake, when material donations to the hospital increased drastically. The issue of coordination, which appeared so prominently in the discourses of my informants, became an even more visible theme as the number and provenance of international actors carrying out interventions increased after the earthquake (Hopmeier et al. 2010). Finally, the issues of obligation and responsibilities remained salient—particularly in regard to the role of Haitian medical professionals and Haitian medical institutions—as the earthquake prompted both departures by Haitian medical staff who felt overwhelmed by the magnitude of the catastrophe, as well as returns to Haiti by members of the diaspora who felt compelled to help their homeland and were able to secure employment through one of the many international initiatives responding to the disaster.

Several months after the earthquake, the closure of private Haitian hospitals and clinics became an issue of concern for Haitian medical professionals and was described repeatedly in the Haitian press. According to standard accounts, the influx of free medical services, treatments, and supplies from international actors had created a climate in which Haitian clinical establishments could not compete and were forced to close. Their staff described with irony how they had opened their doors to all needy patients in the period immediately following the quake, and how, in some cases, international bodies had used private medical facilities with what seemed to the Haitian professionals to represent a tacit understanding that the latter would be compensated for their efforts or receive resources necessary to continue to function after the initial response (*Le Nouvelliste* 2010). In addition, reports suggested that medical professionals were leaving Haiti's public health care system to seek more lucrative positions with international aid agencies (Batha 2011), which had long been described as an internal brain drain.

While it is true that patients in Haiti have often chosen to seek out care from foreigners because it is cheaper than services offered by private clinicians or considered more potent or prestigious because it comes from abroad, it seems unlikely that free care from foreigners was the single or only reason that caused private health facilities to go out of business. Colleagues in Haiti pointed out that the patients who would stand in line in a tent camp to wait for primary health care are not generally those who would have sought out or been able to pay for private health services before the earthquake. Rather, these middle- and upper-class individuals were among those most likely and able to migrate abroad after the quake, if not to North America, then at least to the neighboring Dominican Republic. While the provision of free health services by international bodies may have contributed somewhat to a reduced clientele for Haitian medical professionals in private establishments, it was certainly not the only factor. The fact that it was widely perceived to be the primary cause of closures, however, highlights the tensions and ambivalence that exists between international and local biomedical practitioners in Haiti.

After the earthquake, hundreds of thousands of Haitians found themselves homeless. Those with the possibilities and resources to rebuild began doing so, but, for many more, their only option was to set up in one of the many tent camps that mushroomed throughout the capital, either living in tents sent from abroad by family in the diaspora or international relief organizations, or cobbling together crude shelters from sheets, plastic tarps, cardboard, and any other available scraps of material. These camps lacked the most basic infrastructure and sanitation, and, while relief agencies made efforts to provide clean drinking water and latrines, epidemiologists predicted that the camps' residents were at risk of contracting and propagating infectious diseases.

When a cholera outbreak was signaled in the fall of 2010, it appeared in an unlikely area. Rather than emerging out of the camps, the first cases appeared in the country's Central Plateau. The number of cases quickly multiplied from several dozen to hundreds, then thousands. Local clinics and hospitals were completely overwhelmed, with patients dying of dehydration due to violent diarrhea and vomiting on clinic floors and in hospital yards for lack of beds. As in the case of the earthquake, the exact number of cholera cases and deaths will never be known since many cases of infectious disease are never reported in Haiti, and the country's epidemiological surveillance mechanisms confront a lack of staff and resources even in the best of times.

Initially, the outbreak's origin was a source of debate. Journalists alternately reported that cholera had not been present in Haiti for decades (BBC 2010) or that it had never been documented in the country (CBS 2010). Attention soon turned to a Nepalese MINUSTAH base in the area where the outbreaks occurred, where journalists found that sewage and waste water from the base appeared to be contaminating the local Meille River, which feeds into the Artibonite (Geffrard 2010). Commentators noted that cholera is endemic in Nepal, and that a contingent of Nepalese soldiers had arrived in Haiti following an outbreak of the disease in their home country. As *Vibrio cholerae* can live in and be transmitted by asymptomatic hosts, the UN's claims that its soldiers manifested no signs of the disease carried little weight among critical observers. During the days that followed the identification of the MINUSTAH base as a potential source of contamination,

WHO officials minimized the importance of identifying the outbreak's origins (Jordans 2010). Haitians, particularly sensitive to being repeatedly identified as a source of disease, were outraged, and took public action against the UN and its soldiers. In Cap-Haïtien and other cities around the country, demonstrators, both peaceful and violent, expressed their dismay and fury at the situation.

Several years after it began, the number of deaths attributed to the cholera epidemic was estimated at approximately 9,500, with over 800,000 reported infections (PAHO/WHO 2017). Epidemiologists suspect that cholera may remain an endemic condition in Haiti. While mobilizing impressive sums of foreign aid, materials, and personnel, the medical response to the cholera outbreak has been less spectacular and, as a consequence, less visible in the international media than the aid that followed the earthquake. Not only is the spread of an infectious disease less dramatic than the sudden collapse of thousands of buildings but the work of international workers and volunteers could also be portrayed much more compellingly when they were shown digging for survivors under rubble than distributing chlorine tablets and planning water distribution routes.

As in the case of the earthquake, the cholera outbreak in Haiti and international responses reaffirmed many of the findings and conclusions I had reached prior to it. The epidemic brought into relief the suspicions about what foreigners bring to Haiti, in this case a deadly bacterium. In comparing responses to the earthquake and the cholera epidemic, one returns to a long-standing tension between prioritizing emergency clinical interventions or long-lasting developments in infrastructure as preventive measures against disease outbreaks. While not as numerous as respondents to the earthquake and its aftermath, the number, scope, and diversity of actors and agencies intervening in the context of the cholera outbreak was overwhelming, and coordination continued to be a complex and contentious issue, particularly in controlling a fast-spreading disease that requires various levels of diagnostic, therapeutic, and logistical interventions.

The earthquake and cholera epidemic, therefore, rather than completely reconfiguring the landscape of international medical aid, have amplified and exacerbated preexisting tendencies and patterns. That being said, both of these events have had an important impact on the medical landscape in Haiti. The earthquake represents an event of unprecedented scope for Haiti, in terms of number of sudden deaths, damage to infrastructure, and the destruction and disruption of Haitian institutions. Response to the earthquake was also unprecedented, and highlighted the emergence of new forms of visibility and fundraising, such as donations by cell phone text message and through internet networking sites. The cholera emergency in Haiti had already had major consequences for the country's national stability, in particular given that the UN force assigned to stabilize the country was responsible for introducing the pathogen and for

MINUSTAH's presence in the country. The events of 2010 and 2011 led to the postponement of national elections, given the massive displacements of populations and discrepancies in voter lists at polling stations. Even though postponed, the elections were marred by accusations of fraud at all levels, including pressures by international authorities at the highest levels (Seitenfus 2015). In what is a troubling sign for democratic processes in Haiti, voter turnout has declined significantly in recent elections, in which less than 20 percent of the eligible electorate participated (Johnston 2016). Given that the destiny of Haiti's population is tied up in the confidence and vision of its citizens, a withdrawal from this form of civic participation is worrisome to say the least.

I am frequently asked by North American friends and colleagues if Haiti would be better off without aid. I am never certain how to answer this question; while I appreciate the initial effort to interrogate the efficacy of aid, it is not a serious proposition. International aid to Haiti is not a single phenomenon. It ranges from bilateral development programs to small NGOs, from the philanthropic branches of large corporations to the remittances from relatives living abroad. As shown in this book, its forms are material, intangible, and financial, and it permeates all spheres of life in Haiti. The question about stopping aid to Haiti disregards the country's deep enmeshment in far-reaching structures of commercial and political exchanges. It reflects an impatience with progressive changes, the idea that a tabula rasa would give the opportunity for a fresh start. I remember my horror at being asked by a Canadian university student, "I know I shouldn't say this, but wouldn't they be better off if we just dropped a nuclear bomb on the place?" Part of what made his statement so disturbing was the realization that many other individuals might have similar thoughts but refrain from expressing them. Three days after the earthquake, I met with a group of Haitian university students in Montreal. One young woman, having lost relatives, friends, and her childhood home in the quake, smiled as she spoke through her tears: "My friends and I always used to say that it would be best if Port-au-Prince were totally bulldozed so that we could start over. It looks like we got what we wanted!" So much is expressed through this dark humor: frustration at a sprawling city whose scope and complexity had grown to the point that it seemed more suitable for razing and resurrection than for reform, regret for having expressed the unthinkable, and a sliver of hope that the catastrophe might mark a new beginning. For both the Canadian and the Haitian students, while coming from different backgrounds and with very different stakes in the country's destiny, Haiti's future cannot be imagined under current conditions. Today, over twelve years after the earthquake, many parts of Port-au-Prince have changed little. Residents rebuilt their homes with the same materials as the previous ones. Certain tent camps were destroyed, while others slowly transitioned into more permanent settlements. In the medical domain, the country continues to receive diverse forms of medical collaborations, from short-term medical missions to long-standing medical training programs. It often feels as though little has changed, showing the extent to which global inequalities are deeply embedded in entrenched systems.

Yet there are reasons for optimism when one considers that, as I stated in the introduction to this book, many of the basic demographic indicators used to measure a population's health are improving in Haiti. As this book is going to press, the COVID-19 pandemic has proved to be surprisingly benign in Haiti. The first recorded case in the country was in March 2020, imported by a foreign volunteer at an orphanage. Other cases soon followed, including those brought by Haitian Americans visiting from the United States. Haitians and foreigners predicted that Haiti's population could be devastated by the pandemic. With so many people living and working in crowded conditions, social distancing would be difficult to achieve, and resources such as masks, soap, disinfectant, and water for handwashing would be difficult to procure. Surprisingly, even though testing capacities are quite limited, there do not seem to be widespread symptomatic cases. As of the spring of 2022, the Haitian government has confirmed 30,000 positive cases and fewer than 1,000 fatalities; if the number of serious cases were significantly higher, reports would undoubtedly find their way onto social media. Although some are fearful that variants or subsequent waves could cause greater morbidity and mortality, for the time being, the relative youth of Haiti's population may be offering it protection against a virus that saves its worst consequences for the elderly.

There are other reasons for optimism in Haiti, despite that country's numerous and ongoing challenges (including the assassination of President Jovenel Moïse in July 2021, a catastrophic earthquake in the south of the country in 2021, and ongoing economic hardships). Long-term improvements in a number of other areas, including literacy and the environment (recent studies indicate that rates of deforestation were significantly lower than previously thought, calling into question deeply entrenched narratives about the totality of Haiti as an environmental wasteland). Haitian nursing and medical schools continue to attract and train some of the brightest students in the country, who have struggled and sacrificed enormously to reach that level of educational achievement. While rates of professional emigration are often cited as being higher than 85 percent, two-thirds of the medical residents I interviewed remain in Haiti ten years after I met them, despite nearly all of them saying that they intended to leave the country. Those who continue to work in Haiti do so in a variety of capacities: in private clinics, for international NGOs, and in the public system. While some may consider their nondeparture to be a failure, however, they add to the number of Haitian health professionals who, in the face of countless obstacles, continue to work where they are needed.

Notes

INTRODUCTION

1. Names and specific characteristics of individuals have been changed to protect their privacy.

2. "Don't worry," my Haitian friends told me, "they say that about any foreigner who goes around asking questions." They told me that, after two police officers were assigned to the hospital as part of a Canadian program to provide legal assistance for victims of gender-based violence, rumors circulated that they had in fact been sent by the Haitian government to spy on the hospital's staff.

3. The Cubans at the hospital referred me to their local *jefe de brigada* (brigade chief), who referred me to the national leader of the Cuban mission in Port-au-Prince, who said that he would not have any problem with my interviewing members of the Cuban brigades, but would need approval from authorities in Cuba. When I wrote to him subsequently, I received the following response: "The position of the directors of the Cuban Medical Collaboration is to avoid participating in this type of project, as our collaborators must focus their attention only on the provision of medical aid to the Haitian population" (my translation). Anthropologists conducting fieldwork in Cuba itself have had more success in studying Cuban international medical aid; see Feinsilver 2010 and Brotherton 2013.

4. The hospital was founded as a Catholic institution, and has a chaplain and functional chapel to this day. The hospital's administration, however, is no longer formally tied to the Catholic Church, and the chaplain plays only a very minimal role in the Justinien's everyday activities. During the totality of my fieldwork, I never saw him anywhere other than in his private quarters, located directly behind the hospital's rear courtyard.

1. THE LOGIC OF UNCOORDINATION

1. Calls for increased coordination of aid during this period were not specific to Haiti; in 1991 the UN formed its Office for the Coordination of Humanitarian Affairs.

2. There are exceptions to this model. Among them are the Cuban medical brigades, which send hundreds of medical professionals to Haiti for two-year periods, and long-term North American Christian missionaries. Foreign Catholic missionary clergy have typically lived in Haiti for several decades, although this group is decreasing in size due to aging and death. There are a small number of American Protestant missionary families living in the Cap-Haïtien area, generally involved in running orphanages and schools.

3. Tardiness by Haitians is a common topic of comment and humor by internationals in that country. As in other settings, terms such as *Haitian time* or *island time* imply an inherent disjuncture between one's own notion of time and that of an often racialized, localized other. These comments do not take into account the structural and material constraints that conflict with a strict adherence to a preestablished schedule: bad roads, traffic, vehicle breakdowns, and various types of urgent situations and emergencies related to resource scarcity. During the years I have worked in Haiti, I have noticed the impact cellular phones have had on scheduling. Not only do the phones tell time but they also permit one to inform others of delays and allow for rescheduling.

4. At times a single physician or nurse will travel to or live in Haiti alone to dispense medical care. They are often affiliated, however, with a Haitian institution such as a church or private health establishment.

5. "Gwo nèg yo pa jwi kòb yo ann Ayiti" (Big shots don't enjoy their money in Haiti), I was told on more than one occasion.

6. Poorer Haitians were also targeted, and held for ransoms as little as one hundred US dollars. The kidnapping and murder of twenty-two-year-old Évelyne Sincère, a high school student, and five-year-old Olsmina Jean-Méus, the daughter of a peanut vendor, in 2020 and 2021 are examples of cases in which the victims' families were unable to pay the requested ransom. Both cases received extensive media coverage in Haiti and its diaspora, causing widespread fear and outrage.

7. In addition to influencing relationships with foreign donors, personal appearance and displays of resources are also subject to local codes of self-presentation in Haiti. As in all settings, dress, language, demeanor, and access to visible resources such as vehicles or exclusive spaces convey information about status, worth, and social position in Haiti, but with codes and aesthetics that are both shaped by international influences and distinct from them. Many of my foreign informants often expressed their surprise at the elegance and neatness of Haitians' dress, assuming that high standards for personal appearance in an impoverished country would be inexistent or impossible to achieve.

8. This issue became a central concern in the public distribution of food and other resources after the January 2010 earthquake. Donors developed various strategies to avoid chaos or violence, such as issuing tokens or cards in advance, or by only allowing women to claim resources or behalf of their families. While media reports focused on incidents of postquake violence and looting, reports from colleagues and friends in the area suggest that most distributions were peaceful and orderly.

9. Coverage of Haitians eating cakes made of clay (usually referred to as "mud"), which may also contain margarine and salt, appear from time to time in the North American media. These reports often neglect to mention that Haitians, like other populations, have long consumed clay for its medicinal properties. The sensationalized reports often do not describe the clay's source, preparation, or dosage among those who consume it, and while the cakes' preparation and sale may indeed be related to widespread hunger and malnutrition in Haiti, these reports also perpetuate a legacy of portrayals of poor people of color as less than human, as evidenced by their consumption of nonfood substances (Sites 2006; Associated Press 2008).

10. I use the group's own spelling of its name.

11. Since the initial meetings, there has been a greater effort to include MSPP representatives in the network's activities, and the ministry's local director recently gave a presentation on the process through which foreign NGOs must register for official recognition.

2. "WORKING TOGETHER FOR HEALTH" AT THE HÔPITAL UNIVERSITAIRE JUSTINIEN

1. The term *konbit* refers to a traditional system of exchanging labor in rural Haiti, where peasants form groups to aid members with arduous agricultural work such as clearing land or plowing. *Sante* is the Creole word for health: the group translates its name as meaning "Working Together for Health." Creole names are popular among many international aid groups working in Haiti, whereas Haitian organizations often choose lengthy French names, which are generally shorted to acronyms.

2. The twelve departments are as follows: Anesthesia, the Emergency and Critical Care Unit, Family Medicine, Internal Medicine, Obstetrics and Gynecology, Odontology, Optometry, Orthopedics, Otorhinolaryngology, Pediatrics, Surgery, and Urology.

3. I heard various reasons for the original demise of the washing machine, including pressure from the laundresses, who feared losing their positions and salaries, the unreliability of the hospital's power and water supply, and fears by hospital staff that the machine was incapable of thoroughly cleaning blood-stained surgical drapes and gowns. Aid failures, which often stem from multiple causes, frequently generate competing narratives and moral claims to determine their "true" root causes and to attribute blame.

4. This type of aid is common at the Hôpital Sacré-Coeur in the city of Milot, a private Catholic hospital located twelve kilometers from Cap-Haïtien. This hospital receives between twenty and thirty teams a year for weeklong stays, including specialists in cardiology, orthopedics, urology, and others. Most teams come from the United States, make an annual visit to the hospital, and stay in a nearby compound. Teams often carry out complex or specialized procedures that are not normally available in northern Haiti. The hospital's full-time staff screens patients throughout the year to identify patients that would benefit from these procedures.

5. During my research, the Justinien received only one team carrying out regular, short-term clinical interventions: an orthopedic surgeon employed by CURE International (a North American NGO) and based in Santo Domingo traveled to Cap-Haïtien every three months to carry out orthopedic surgeries. Accompanied by Dominican and North American physicians, nurses, and technicians, he would recruit and select patients on the first days of his trip, and over the following four or five days he would carry out a high number of surgeries, operating as many as twenty hours per day.

6. These children may eventually be referred to local orphanages, be adopted into a family seeking a child, or face lives of forced domestic servitude (the infamous Haitian category of *restavèk*) and other forms of exploitation.

7. Infants' parents or relatives are still required to purchase tanks of oxygen from a vendor outside the hospital.

8. In a growing number of cases, the Justinien staff has approached Konbit Sante about initiating a partnership. While visiting Konbit Sante staff and volunteers are regularly solicited for different forms of immediate and often individual aid, they are more inclined to respond positively to proposals for institutional partnerships with structured programs.

9. *Mis* is both the word for nurse and the title used to address nurses. The term's origin reflects the influence of the 1915–34 US Marine occupation, which brought modern nursing as an occupation to Haiti.

10. The Konbit Sante nurses never expressed this idea. I believe they interpreted the Haitian nurses' suspicion not as a questioning of their motivations, but rather as skepticism that changes were possible.

11. With the undermining of Haiti's agricultural sector by neoliberal trade policies and limited opportunities in construction, skilled trades, or the service sector, work unloading containers and delivering goods (often subsidized agricultural products or donated secondhand goods from abroad) in wheelbarrows represents one of the few remaining income-generating activities available to men in Haiti. The physical toll of this type of work (hernias, sprains, accidents, etc.) are significant.

12. Deforestation, erosion, and unpaved roads contribute to a major dust problem throughout Haiti, and even objects stored in closed spaces are quickly covered with a thick layer of grime.

13. Informants were wary of pointing to specific instances of aid that was diverted or misappropriated; they were more likely to generalize about most cases of aid. One common complaint was that a great deal of aid funds are spent on expensive and useless *séminaires*, trainings or workshops, which were held at exclusive hotels in Port-au-Prince or at beach resorts.

14. Direct Relief International is such an organization that is active at the HUJ. The group's main purpose is to provide medical supplies to health institutions in impoverished settings.

15. *Don* ("donation" or "gift" in both French and Creole) was used by Haitian informants. At times, the Creole term *kado* (from the French *cadeau*, or "present") was also used.

16. His departure from Haiti and his job with Konbit Sante were fairly abrupt. Although he had maintained good relationships with his employers, tension emerged in the final months related to his expectations and hopes that Konbit Sante would continue to pay his salary even after his departure. Dr. Gilles had come to think of Konbit Sante as a source of sustained personal support, while the organization was unwilling or unable to modify its budget to pay a former employee.

3. BETWEEN A FUND AND A HARD PLACE

1. Checks are sometimes still issued in the name of the deceased person, earning them the moniker *chèk zonbi* (zombie checks).

2. Two residents refused to be interviewed: one who repeatedly missed appointments I set with him, and another who simply told me that she did not wish to answer any of my questions. As many of the residents themselves had to conduct qualitative interviews as part of their own required research projects, most were already familiar with the interview process.

3. I was unable to determine why a graduate of the state university came to a residency at the Justinien: the resident in question would not answer my direct questions about the situation.

4. Five of the residents at the Justinien had domestic employees working for them as cooks, laundresses, and nannies at the hospital.

5. The residents' protest was reminiscent of *bat tenèb*, or "beating the darkness," a form of protest in poor urban areas that was used during coup d'états and other periods of political repression (Maternowska 2006, 7). During bat tenèb, participants beat metal items such as pots, pans, and metal posts to create a din of collective protest.

6. The word *klowòks* became popular throughout Haiti in the spring of 2008 when rising food prices led to hunger and protests throughout the country. The term comes from the commercial brand of bleach Clorox, and referred to the burning sensation in the belly caused by extreme hunger.

7. Brain gain has also been used to describe the effect of migrating professionals to a wealthier country.

8. The quantity of remittances sent to overseas migrants is difficult to estimate, as these often do not pass through official channels. The importance of international aid in relation to other forms of revenue may increase as a result of the January 2010 earthquake, however funds disbursed are often less than those officially pledged, and are often used for expenses outside of Haiti, such as imported materials or salaries for foreign experts.

4. COMPONENTS OF A MORAL ECONOMY

1. Brodwin (1996) and Brown ([1991] 2001) also provide insightful analyses of how morality, economics, and diverse forms of healing overlap in Haiti and in the Haitian diaspora.

2. Fassin offers his definition, which he bases on Jean-Baptiste Say's early nineteenth-century definition of political economy: "the production, distribution, circulation, and utilization of moral sentiments, emotions and values, norms, and obligations in the social

realm" (2009, 1257, my translation). Fassin specifies that this usage highlights "moral" over "economy"; brings together norms, values, and emotions; and can be applied to society as a whole and all social worlds. Unlike Fassin, I include the movement of material goods, funds, labor, and other resources in my analysis, given their importance in settings such as Haiti, where many of the sentiments, values, and norms circulating in this sphere are inextricably linked to tangible resources.

3. See, for example, O'Brien and Gostin 2011. WHO's *World Health Report 2006* focused on the global health workforce, and the Global Health Workforce Alliance was created in the same year.

4. A medical resident told me that once a year, he would receive patients claiming to have received hernia surgeries from a group of visiting foreign health workers. He said, "The way that those procedures were done, you can tell that they weren't surgeons. Maybe they were students, or maybe they were trying out something new."

5. I did not hear people speak of "general interest" as the opposite of "personal interest." Instead, the term *dezenterese* (disinterested) was used to describe altruistic actions that were carried out without any thought of personal gain or advancement. The most disinterested acts were toward complete strangers, as the most obvious interests to be nourished through aid and gifts were interpersonal relationships and the opportunities they offered for reciprocal exchanges. The idea that gestures or gifts directed toward strangers constitute a superior class of transactions appears in a variety of ethical traditions, from the Hindu concept of *dān* (Bornstein 2012) to Maimonides's ranking of gifts to the biblical parable of the Good Samaritan.

6. The figure was brought to prominence by President Jean-Bertrand Aristide during his second term in office in 2003 (Charles 2003). Prior to his 2015 visit to Haiti, the French premier François Hollande claimed that he would settle France's debt to Haiti, which prompted rekindled speculation about the return of the sum extorted from the newly independent republic. Members of his cabinet were quick to specify that the debt in question was moral, not financial.

7. In the late 1700s, a force of over five hundred *hommes libres de couleur* (free men of color) from Saint-Domingue joined American forces in battles against the British in Savannah, Georgia (Garrigus 1992).

8. These sentiments, while widespread in Haiti's diaspora, are not uncontested or uncomplicated: a Haitian American physician recounted hearing from his aunt that, to her, Haiti was like a rotten limb, one that she had amputated after arriving in the United States.

9. In this way, medical aid resembles the gift of blood as described by Richard Titmuss (1997), a gift that the giver does not expect or hope to receive in return.

5. SAINTS, VILLAINS, AND CHAMPIONS

1. The few published critiques of Farmer and his work focus on his ties to Bill Clinton and the United Nations, or accuse him of being complicit with dominant economic and political structures. See Herz 2013 and Dubal 2012.

2. Although Albert Schweitzer never traveled to Haiti, his work had a decisive influence on Larimer Mellon, an American physician and philanthropist who, with his wife Gwen Mellon, established the Hôpital Albert Schweitzer (HAS), a major hospital and health network in central Haiti that, until recently, was the most famous hospital in the country. Mellon and Schweitzer corresponded extensively over the course of nearly twenty years (Byers 1996), and Schweitzer's legacy on the hospital today is still palpable, ranging from the institution's ever-present motto of "Reverence for Life" to the continued presence of French, German, and Swiss staff and volunteers inspired by Schweitzer's legacy. A vignette

in Kidder's biography recounts a negative experience of Farmer's during his visit to the HAS on his first trip to Haiti: "He had high expectations, and it was a good-looking hospital, he thought. But it was staffed mainly by white, expatriate doctors. He'd imagined something different—a hospital at least partly devoted to training Haitians. Besides, the Schweitzer didn't have a job for him just then, in spite of his Mellon contact. He went back to the city, feeling, he'd say, 'deflated'" (Kidder 2003, 65). HAS cannot be considered a Haitian extension of Albert Schweitzer's African work—Schweitzer was not officially affiliated with the hospital. The story is indicative, however, of Farmer's dissatisfaction with the forms of international medical aid he found in Haiti. It also hints at some of the measures he would take to correct what he perceived to be failings in other establishments.

References

Adams, Vincanne. 2016. *Metrics: What Counts in Global Health*. Durham, NC: Duke University Press.

Associated Press. 2008. "Haiti's Poor Resort to Eating Mud as Prices Rise." Accessed September 29, 2019. https://www.nbcnews.com/id/wbna22902512.

Ballard, C. M. 1965. "Albert Schweitzer." *Contemporary Review* 207:225.

Batha, Emma. 2011. "Haiti Loses Its Doctors and Nurses to Aid Groups." Accessed May 29, 2019. Alertnet. https://news.trust.org/item/20110114184700-maqot?view=print.

BBC. 2010. "Haiti Cholera: UN Peacekeepers to Blame, Report Says." Accessed August 19, 2020. http://www.bbc.co.uk/news/world-latin-america-11943902.

Beckett, Greg. 2008. "The End of Haiti: History under Conditions of Impossibility." PhD diss., University of Chicago.

———. 2019. *There Is No More Haiti: Between Life and Death in Port-au-Prince*. Oakland, CA: University of California Press.

Benton, Adia. 2015. *HIV Exceptionalism: Development through Disease in Sierra Leone*. Minneapolis: University of Minnesota Press.

Bhargavan, Alok, Frédéric Docquier, and Yasser Moullan. 2011. "Modeling the Effect of Physician Emigration on Human Development." *Economics and Human Biology* 9 (2): 172–83.

Bordes, Ary. 1992. *Médecine et santé publique en Haïti: Période de l'occupation américaine, 1915–1934*. Port-au-Prince: Henri Deschamps.

———. 1997. *La Santé de la République, 1934–1957*. Port-au-Prince: Henri Deschamps.

Bornstein, Erica. 2005. *The Spirit of Development: Protestant NGOs, Morality and Economics in Zimbabwe*. London: Routledge.

———. 2010. "The Value of Orphans." In *Forces of Compassion: Humanitarianism between Ethics and Politics*, edited by Erica Bornstein and Peter Redfield, 123–47. Santa Fe, NM: SAR Press.

———. 2012. *Disquieting Gifts: Humanitarianism in New Delhi*. Palo Alto, CA: Stanford University Press.

Brada, Betsey. 2010. "'Not Here': Making the Space and Subjects of 'Global Health' in Botswana." *Culture, Medicine and Psychiatry* 35:285–312.

Brodwin, Paul. 1996. *Medicine and Morality in Haiti: The Contest for Healing Power*. Cambridge: Cambridge University Press.

Brotherton, P. Sean. 2013. "Fueling la Revolución: Itinerant Physicians, Transactional Humanitarianism, and Shifting Moral Economies." In *Health Travels: Cuban Health(Care) on the Island and around the World*, edited by Nancy Burke, 127–51. San Francisco: University of California Medical Humanities Consortium.

Brown, Karen McCarthy. [1991] 2001. *Mama Lola: A Vodou Priestess in Brooklyn*. 2nd ed. Berkeley: University of California Press.

Brown, Theodore, Marcus Cueto, and Elizabeth Fee. 2006. "The World Health Organization and the Transition from 'International' to 'Global.'" *American Journal of Public Health* 96 (1): 62–72.

Buss, Terry. 2008. *Haiti in the Balance: Why Foreign Aid Has Failed and What We Can Do About It*. Washington, DC: Brookings Institution Press.

Butt, Leslie. 2002. "The Suffering Stranger: Medical Anthropology and International Morality." *Medical Anthropology* 21 (1): 1–24.

Byers, Jeannette. 1996. *Brothers in Spirit: The Correspondence of Albert Schweitzer and William Larimer Mellon, Jr.* Syracuse, NY: Syracuse University Press.

Canadian AIDS Treatment Information Exchange. 2018. "The Epidemiology of HIV in Canada." Accessed February 4, 2018. http://www.catie.ca/en/fact-sheets/epidemiology/epidemiology-hiv-canada.

Carruth, Lauren. 2021. *Love and Liberation: Humanitarian Work in Ethiopia's Somali Region*. Ithaca, NY: Cornell University Press.

Castor, Suzy. 1988. *L'Occupation américaine d'Haïti*. Port-au-Prince: CRESFED.

CBS. 2010. "Haiti's Cholera Death Count Passes 1000." Accessed November 16, 2019. https://www.cbsnews.com/news/haitis-cholera-death-count-passes-1000/.

Central Intelligence Agency. 2018. "World Factbook." Accessed January 23, 2018. https://www.cia.gov/library/publications/the-world-factbook/rankorder/2155rank.html.

Charles, Jacqueline. 2003. "Aristide Pushes for Reparations from France." *Miami Herald*, December 18, 2003. Accessed July 22, 2020. http://www.latinamericanstudies.org/haiti/haiti-restitution.htm.

CIDA. 2009. "Minister Oda Concludes a Successful Visit to Haiti: Ensuring That Canadian Assistance in Haiti Is Well-Directed and Effective." Accessed June 24, 2010. http://www.acdi-cida.gc.ca/acdi-cida/ACDI-CIDA.nsf/eng/NAT-31714416-PWR.

Clinton, William J. 2007. *Giving: How Each of Us Can Change the World*. New York: Alfred A. Knopf.

Cole, Teju. 2012. "The White Savior-Industrial Complex." *Atlantic*, March 21, 2012. Accessed January 19, 2016. https://www.theatlantic.com/international/archive/2012/03/the-white-savior-industrial-complex/254843/.

Constant, André. 1967. *L'Hôpital Justinien du Cap-Haïtien*. Port-au-Prince: Presses Nationales d'Haïti.

Cousins, Norman. 1960. *Dr. Schweitzer of Lambaréné*. New York: Harper and Brothers.

Crane, Johanna Tayloe. 2013. *Scrambling for Africa: AIDS, Expertise, and the Rise of American Global Health Science*. Ithaca, NY: Cornell University Press.

Cueto, Marcos. 1994a. Introduction to *Missionaries of Science: The Rockefeller Foundation and Latin America*, edited by Marcos Cueto, iv–xx. Bloomington: Indiana University Press.

——. 1994b. "Visions of Science and Development: The Rockefeller Foundation's Latin American Surveys of the 1920s." In *Missionaries of Science: The Rockefeller Foundation and Latin America*, edited by Marcos Cueto, 1–22. Bloomington: Indiana University Press.

Dahl, Bianca. 2015. "Sexy Orphans and Sugar Daddies: The Sexual and Moral Politics of Aid for AIDS in Botswana." *Comparative International Development* 50 (4). Accessed August 19, 2017. https://doi.org/10.1007/s12116-015-9195-1.

Danticat, Edwidge. [2007] 2008. *Brother, I'm Dying*. 2nd ed. New York: Vintage Books.

de Waal, Alex. 1997. *Famine Crimes: Politics and the Disaster Relief Industry in Africa*. Bloomington: Indiana University Press.

Dubal, Sam. 2012. "Renouncing Paul Farmer." May 27, 2012. Accessed May 14, 2013. http://samdubal.blogspot.com/2012/05/renouncing-paul-farmer-desperate-plea.html.

Dubois, Carl-Ardy, France Brunelle, and Carine Rousseau. 2007. *Analyses et projection: Recensement des ressources humaines en santé en Haïti*. Technical Report. Montreal: Project PARC, Unité de Santé Internationale, Université de Montréal.

Dubois, Laurent. 2004. *Avengers of the New World: The Story of the Haitian Revolution*. Cambridge, MA: Harvard University Press.

Easterly, William. 2006. *The White Man's Burden: Why the West's Efforts to Aid the Rest Have Done So Much Ill and So Little Good*. New York: Penguin Books.

Edelman, Mark. 2005. "Bringing the Moral Economy Back In . . . to the Study of 21st-Century Transnational Peasant Movements." *American Anthropologist* 107 (3): 331–45.

Fagen, Patricia Weiss. 2009. "Haitian Diasporic Associations and Their Investments in Basic Social Services in Haiti." Report prepared for the Inter-American Development Bank. Accessed January 14, 2011. http://www12.georgetown.edu/sfs/isim/Publications/PatPubs/Haitian%20Diapora%20Associations.pdf.

Farmer, Paul. 1988. "Bad Blood, Spoiled Milk: Bodily Fluids as Moral Barometers in Rural Haiti." *American Ethnologist* 15 (1): 62–83.

——. 1992. *AIDS and Accusation: Haiti and the Geography of Blame*. Berkeley: University of California Press.

——. 1999. *Infections and Inequalities: The New Plagues*. Berkeley: University of California Press.

——. 2003. *Pathologies of Power: Health, Human Rights, and the New War on the Poor*. Berkeley: University of California Press.

——. 2011. *Haiti after the Earthquake*. New York: PublicAffairs.

——. 2020. *Fevers, Feuds and Diamonds: Ebola and the Ravages of History*. New York: Farrar, Straus and Giroux.

Fassin, Didier. 2009. "Les économies morales revisitées: Étude critique suivie de quelques propositions." *Annales. Histoire, Sciences Sociales* 64 (6): 1237–66.

Fatton, Robert. 2002. *Haiti's Predatory Republic: The Unending Transition to Democracy*. Boulder, CO: Lynne Rienner.

Feinsilver, Julie M. 2010. "Fifty Years of Cuba's Medical Diplomacy: From Idealism to Pragmatism." *Cuban Studies* 41:85–104.

Fisher, Sybille. 2004. *Modernity Disavowed: Haiti and the Cultures of Slavery in the Age of Revolution*. Durham, NC: Duke University Press.

Foreign and Commonwealth Office. 2009. "Travel and Living Abroad: Haiti." Accessed August 29, 2011. http://www.fco.gov.uk.

Foster, Charles R., and Albert Valdman, eds. 1984. *Haiti—Today and Tomorrow: An Interdisciplinary Study*. Lanham, MD: University Press of America.

Fourie, Willem. 2015. "Four Concepts of Africa." *HTS Teologiese Studies/Theological Studies* 71 (3): 1–10.

Garrigus, John. 1992. "Catalyst of Catastrophe? Saint-Domingue's Free Men of Color and the Battle of Savannah, 1779–1782." *Revista/Review Interamericana* 22 (1–2): 109–25.

Geffrard, Robenson. 2010. "Une maladie importée, La MINUSTAH clame son innocence." *Le Nouvelliste*, October 26, 2010. Accessed October 28, 2011. http://lenouvelliste.com/article.php?PubID=&ArticleId=85056.

Giafferi-Dombre, Nadia. 2007. *Une ethnologue à Port-au-Prince*. Paris: L'Harmattan.

Glick Schiller, Nina, and Georges E. Fouron. 2001. *Georges Woke Up Laughing: Long-Distance Nationalism and the Search for Home*. Durham, NC: Duke University Press.

Graeber, David. 2011. *Debt: The First 5,000 Years*. Brooklyn, NY: Melville House.

Griffith, David. 2009. "The Moral Economy of Tobacco." *American Anthropologist* 111 (4): 432–42.

Grubel, Herbert, and Anthony Scott. 1977. *The Brain Drain: Determinant, Measurement and Welfare Effects.* Waterloo: Wilfrid Laurier University Press.

Hancock, Graham. 1994. *The Lords of Poverty: The Power, Prestige, and Corruption of the International Aid Business.* New York: Atlantic Monthly Press.

Hefferan, Tara. 2007. *Twinning Faith and Development: Catholic Parish Partnership in the US and Haiti.* West Hartford, CT: Kumarian Press.

Herz, Ansel. 2013. "The Uses of Paul Farmer." *Counterpunch.* January 17, 2013. Accessed September 29, 2015. https://www.counterpunch.org/2013/01/17/the-uses-of-paul-farmer/.

Hoffman, Léon-François. 1984. "Francophilia and Cultural Nationalism in Haiti." In Foster and Valdman 1984, 57–76.

Honoré, Jean G., Jean G. Balan, Gabriel Thymothé, Joanna Diallo, and Scott Barnhart. 2016. "Instability Adversely Affects HIV Care in Haiti." *Lancet* 388 (10054): 1877. Accessed November 2, 2017. https://doi.org/10.1016/S0140-6736(16)31804-9.

Hopmeier, Michael J., Jean William Pape, David Paulison, Richard Carmona, Tim Davis, Kobi Peleg, Gili Shenhar, Colleen Conway-Welch, Sten H. Vermund, Janet Nicotera, Arthur L. Kellermann et al. 2010. "Reflections on the Initial Multinational Response to the Earthquake in Haiti." *Population Health Management* 13 (3): 105–13.

Icart, Jean-Claude. 2004. "Le Québec et Haïti: Une histoire ancienne." *Une histoire à découvrir! Caps-aux-Diamants* 79:30–34. Accessed May 13, 2011. http://id.erudit.org/iderudit/7190ac.

Interim Cooperation Framework. 2006. *ICF Summary Report.* Accessed June 4, 2011. http://haiticci.undg.org/uploads/ReportVersion8%20Eng%20FINAL%20Low%20Res.pdf.

International Monetary Fund. 2009. Press release. IMF and World Bank Approve US$1.2 Billion Debt Relief for Haiti. July 1, 2009. Accessed July 28, 2012. https://www.imf.org/en/News/Articles/2015/09/14/01/49/pr09243.

Institut Haïtien de l'Enfance (IHE) and ICF. 2018. *Haïti: Enquête Mortalité, Morbidité et Utilisation des Services, 2016–2017* (EMMUS–VI). Pétion-Ville and Rockville, MD: IHE and ICF.

James, Erica. 2010. *Democratic Insecurities: Violence, Trauma and Intervention in Haiti.* Berkeley: University of California Press.

Johnston, Jake. 2016. "Breakdown of Preliminary Election Results in Haiti." Center for Economic and Policy Research. Accessed January 30, 2022. https://cepr.net/breakdown-of-preliminary-election-results-in-haiti/.

Jordans, Frank. 2010. "UN Appeals for $164M to Combat Haiti Cholera." Associated Press. Accessed November 12, 2011. ABC News. http://abcnews.go.com/Health/wireStory?id=12129250.

Kidder, Tracy. 2003. *Mountains beyond Mountains: The Quest of Dr. Paul Farmer, a Man Who Would Cure the World.* New York: Random House.

Konbit Sante. n.d. "Get Involved." Accessed March 17, 2014. http://konbitsante.org/get-involved/haiti-volunteers.

Koplan, Jeffrey, T. Christopher Bond, Michael H. Merson, K. Srinath Reddy et al. 2009. "Towards a Common Definition of Global Health." *Lancet* 373:1993–95.

Lakoff, Andrew. 2010. "Two Regimes of Global Health." *Humanity* 1 (1): 59–79.

Le Nouvelliste. 2010. "Les hôpitaux privés entrevoient le bout du tunnel." June 2, 2010. Accessed November 2, 2011. http://www.lenouvelliste.com/article.php?PubID=1&ArticleID=80206.

Lewison, Martin. 1999. "Conflicts of Interest? The Ethics of Usury." *Journal of Business Ethics* 22 (4): 327–39.

MacFarquhar, Neil. 2010. "Haiti Frets over Aid and Control of Rebuilding." *New York Times*, March 31, 2010. Accessed March 30, 2011. http://www.nytimes.com/2010/03/31/world/Americas/31haiti.html.

Maki, Jesse, Munirih Qualls, Benjamin White, Sharon Kleefield, and Robert Crone. 2008. "Health Impact Assessment and Short-Term Medical Missions: A Methods Study to Evaluate Quality of Care." *BMC Health Services Research* 8:121–28.

Malkki, Liisa. 2010. "Children, Humanity and the Infantilization of Peace." In *In the Name of Humanity: The Government of Threat and Care*, edited by Ilana Feldman and Miriam Ticktin, 58–85. Durham, NC: Duke University Press.

——. 2015. *The Need to Help: The Domestic Arts of International Humanitarianism*. Durham, NC: Duke University Press.

Manegold, Catherine. 1994. "Mission to Haiti: The Scene; For Aristide's Followers, Every Step Is a Dance, Every Cheer a Song." *New York Times*, October 16, 1994.

Manzaneda, José. 2010. "Médicos de Cuba en Haití: La solidaridad silenciada." January, 23, 2010. Accessed March 31, 2011. http://www.rebelion.org/noticia.php?id=99129.

Maternowska, M. Catherine. 2006. *Reproducing Inequities: Poverty and the Politics of Population in Haiti*. Piscataway, NJ: Rutgers University Press.

Mattoo, Aaditya, Ileana Cristina Neagu, and Çağlar Özden. 2005. *Brain Waste? Educated Immigrants in the U.S. Labor Market*. World Bank Policy Research Working Paper 3581. Washington, DC: World Bank.

Mauss, Marcel. 1950. "Essai sur le don: Forme et raison de l'échange dans les sociétés archaïques." *L'Année Sociologique* 1:30–186.

McAlister, Elizabeth. 2002. *Rara! Vodou, Power and Performance in Haiti and Its Diaspora*. Berkeley: University of California Press.

——. 2010. "Haiti and the Unseen World." SSRC Blog, The Immanent Frame: Secularism, Religion and the Public Sphere. Accessed May 18, 2011. http://blogs.ssrc.org/tif/2010/01/31/haiti-and-the-unseen-world/.

McKay, Ramah. 2018. *Medicine in the Meantime: The Work of Care in Mozambique*. Durham, NC: Duke University Press.

Mews, Constant J., and Ibrahim Abraham. 2007. "Usury and Just Compensation: Religious and Financial Ethics in Historical Perspective." *Journal of Business Ethics* 72 (1): 1–15.

Mills, Sean. 2016. *A Place in the Sun: Haiti, Haitians, and the Remaking of Quebec*. Montreal: McGill-Queen's University Press.

Ministère de la Planification et de la Cooperation Externe. n.d. Liste actualisée des ong reconnues pour l'exercice fiscal 2015–2016. Accessed December 20, 2021. https://issuu.com/jean-juniorjoseph/docs/liste_des_ong_reconnues.

Minn, Pierre. 2007. "Toward an Anthropology of Humanitarianism." *Journal of Humanitarian Assistance*. August 6, 2007. Accessed August 3, 2010. http://sites.tufts.edu/jha/archives/51.

——. 2010. "Medical Humanitarianism and Health as a Human Right on the Haitian-Dominican Border." In *Haiti and the Haitian Diaspora in the Wider Caribbean*, edited by Philippe Zacaïr, 103–20. Gainesville: University of Florida Press.

——. 2016. "The Tyranny of the Widget: An American Medical Aid Organization's Struggles with Quantification." In *Metrics: What Counts in Global Health*, edited by Vincanne Adams, 203–24. Durham, NC: Duke University Press.

Moreau de Saint-Méry, Médéric Louis Élie. [1789] 1958. *Description topographique, physique, civile, politique et historique de la partie française de l'Isle Saint-Domingue*. Paris: Société de l'Histoire des Colonies Françaises.

Moyo, Dambisa. 2009. *Dead Aid: Why Aid Is Not Working and How There Is a Better Way for Africa*. New York: Farrar, Straus and Giroux.

Muir, Sarah, and Akhil Gupta. 2018. "Rethinking the Anthropology of Corruption: An Introduction to Supplement 18." *Current Anthropology* 59 (Supplement 18): S4–S15.

Nader, Laura. 2011. "Ethnography as Theory." *HAU: Journal of Ethnographic Theory* 1 (1): 211–19.

NPR. 2015. "In Search of the Red Cross' $500 million in Haiti Relief." June 3, 2015. Accessed September 19, 2021. https://www.npr.org/2015/06/03/411524156/in-search-of-the-red-cross-500-million-in-haiti-relief.

O'Brien, Paula, and Lawrence O. Gostin. 2011. "Health Worker Shortages and Global Justice." New York: Milbank Memorial Fund. http://www.milbank.org/uploads/documents/HealthWorkerShortages_Mech/HealthWorkerShortages_Mech.html, accessed October 10, 2013.

OCHA. 2011. "Haiti: One Year Later." Report of the United Nations Office for the Coordination of Humanitarian Affairs. Accessed November 21, 2012. http://ochaonline.un.org/HaitiEarthquakeResponse/tabid/7331/language/en-US/Default.aspx.

Olsen, William C., and Thomas J. Csordas, eds. 2019. *Engaging Evil: A Moral Anthropology*. New York: Berghahn Books.

O'Neill, Sean. 2018. "Oxfam in Haiti: 'It Was Like a Caligula Orgy with Prostitutes in Oxfam T-Shirts.'" *London Times*, February 9, 2018.

Oxfam. 2005. "Kicking Down the Door: How Upcoming WTO Talks Threaten Farmers in Poor Countries." Report. Accessed February 24, 2011. http://www.maketradefair.com/en/assets/english/kickingreport.pdf.

———. 2010. "Haiti Earthquake: What Oxfam Is Doing." Accessed February 24, 2011. http://www.oxfam.org/en/emergencies/haiti-earthquake/what-oxfam-is-doing.

Özden, Çağlar, and Maurice Schiff. 2006. *International Migration, Remittances, and the Brain Drain*. Washington, DC: World Bank and Palgrave Macmillan. Accessed November 5, 2013. https://openknowledge.worldbank.org/handle/10986/6929.

PAHO/WHO. 2017. "Epidemiological Update: Cholera." December 28, 2017. Washington, DC: PAHO/WHO. Accessed February 28, 2018. http://www.paho.org/hq/cholera.

Pandolfi, Mariella. 2002. "'Moral Entrepreneurs,' souverainetés mouvantes et barbelés: Le bio-politique dans les Balkans postcommunistes." *Anthropologie et sociétés* 26 (1): 29–51.

Partners in Health. 2020. *Annual Report 2020*. Accessed April 22, 2021. https://www.pih.org/sites/default/files/pdf/pih-annual-report-2020.pdf?2021.

Patterson, Amy. 2018. *Africa and Global Health Governance: Domestic Politics and International Structures*. Baltimore: Johns Hopkins University Press.

Patterson, Rubin. 2007. "Going around the Drain-Gain Debate with Brain Circulation." In *African Brain Circulation: Beyond the Drain-Gain Debate*, edited by Rubin Patterson, 1–14. Leiden: Koninkrijke Brill NV.

Peebles, Gustav. 2010. "The Anthropology of Credit and Debt." *Annual Review of Anthropology* 39:225–40.

Plummer, Brenda Gayle. 1992. *Haiti and the United States: The Psychological Moment*. Athens: University of Georgia Press.

Portes, Alejandro, and Ramón Grosfoguel. 1994. "Caribbean Diasporas: Migration and Ethnic Communities." *Annals of the American Academy of Political and*

Social Science 533:48–69. Accessed March 3, 2011. http://ann.sagepub.com/content/533/1/48.full.pdf+html.

Ramachandran, Vijaya, and Julie Walz. 2013. "Haiti's Earthquake Generated a $9bn Response—Where Did the Money Go?" *Guardian*, January 14, 2013.

Reagan, Andrew J., Lewis Mitchell, Dilan Kiley, Christopher M. Danforth, and Peter Sheridan Dodds. 2016. "The Emotional Arcs of Stories Are Dominated by Six Basic Shapes." *EPJ Data Science* 5 (31): 1–12.

Redfield, Peter. 2005. "Doctors, Borders and Life in Crisis." *Cultural Anthropology* 20 (3): 328–61.

——. 2013. *Life in Crisis: The Ethical Journey of Doctors Without Borders*. Berkeley: University of California Press.

Rieff, David. 2002. *A Bed for the Night: Humanitarianism in Crisis*. New York: Simon and Schuster.

Robbins, Joel. 2013. "Beyond the Suffering Subject: Toward an Anthropology of the Good." *Journal of the Royal Anthropological Institute* 19 (3): 447–62.

Sahay, Anjali. 2009. *Indian Diaspora in the United States: Brain Drain or Gain?* Lanham, MD: Lexington Books.

Sanders, Grace. 2010. "Third-World Disney: Slumming and Philanthropic Tourism in Pre-Earthquake Port-au-Prince, 1945–1970." Paper presented at the 22nd Annual Meeting of the Haitian Studies Association, Providence, RI, November 11–13, 2010.

Scott, James. 1976. *The Moral Economy of the Peasant: Rebellion and Subsistence in Southeast Asia*. New Haven, CT: Yale University Press.

Seitenfus, Ricardo. 2015. *L'aide internationale en Haïti: Dilemme et égarements*. Montreal and Port-au-Prince: CIDIHCA and Les Presses de l'Université d'État d'Haïti.

Sites, Kevin. 2006. "Haitian Mud Pies: Video." Accessed July 4, 2011. http://new.music.yahoo.com/blogs/blogs/49777/haitian-mud-pies-video/.

Smith, Daniel Jordan. 2008. *A Culture of Corruption: Everyday Deception and Popular Discontent in Nigeria*. Princeton, NJ: Princeton University Press.

Solimano, Andrés. 2008. *The International Mobility of Talent: Types, Causes, and Development Impact*. Oxford: Oxford University Press.

Sontag, Deborah. 2012. "Rebuilding in Haiti Lags after Billions in Post-Quake Aid." *New York Times*, December 23, 2012.

Strathern, Marilyn, ed. 2000. *Audit Cultures: Anthropological Studies in Accountability, Ethics and the Academy*. London: Routledge.

Street, Alice. 2014. *Biomedicine in an Unstable Place: Infrastructure and Personhood in a Papua New Guinean Hospital*. Durham, NC: Duke University Press.

Sykes, Kevin. 2014. "Short-Term Medical Service Trips: A Systematic Review of the Evidence." *American Journal of Public Health* 104 (7): 38–48. Accessed April 30, 2015. http://10.2105/AJPH.2014.301983.

Telesur. 2011. "Venezuela ratifica que continuará apoyo al pueblo de Haití." May 14, 2011. Accessed January 5, 2013. http://exwebserv.telesurtv.net/EN/noticias/92848-NN/venezuela-ratifica-que-continuara-apoyo-al-pueblo-de-haiti/.

Thompson, E. P. 1963. *The Making of the English Working Class*. London: Victor Gollancz.

——. 1971. "The Moral Economy of the English Crowd in the Eighteenth Century." *Past and Present* 50 (1): 76–136.

——. 1991. *Customs in Common*. London: Merlin Press.

Ticktin, Miriam. 2014. "Transnational Humanitarianism." *Annual Review of Anthropology* 43:273–89.

Titmuss, Richard. [1970] 1997. *The Gift Relationship: From Human Blood to Social Policy*. New York: W. W. Norton.

Trouillot, Michel-Rolph. 1990. *Haiti: State against Nation*. New York: Monthly Review Press.

——. 1995. *Silencing the Past: Power and the Production of History*. Boston, MA: Beacon Press.

UN Ad Hoc Advisory Group on Haiti. 1999. "Report of the Ad Hoc Advisory Group on Haiti to the Economic and Social Council." Accessed September 23, 2010. http://www.un.org/esa/documents/ecosoc/docs/1999/e1999-dft8.htm.

UNHCR. 2008. "Haiti: Frequency of Kidnappings for Ransom; Groups Targeted by Kidnappers; Measures Taken by the Authorities to Combat Kidnappings (2004–2007)." Report. Accessed May 19, 2009. http://www.unhcr.org/refworld/country,4804c0e5c,0.html.

Unite for Sight. 2016. "Global Health Course, Module 1: What Are Best Practice 'Gold Standard' Principles?" Accessed July 14, 2017. http://www.uniteforsight.org/global-health-course/module1.

US Department of State. 2010. "Haiti: Background Notes." Accessed April 5, 2011. http://www.state.gov/r/pa/ei/bgn/1982.htm#econ.

Valdman, Albert. 1984. "The Linguistic Situation of Haiti." In Foster and Valdman 1984, 77–100.

——. 2007. *Haitian Creole–English Bilingual Dictionary*. Bloomington: Indiana University Creole Institute.

Weaver, Karol K. 2006. *Medical Revolutionaries: The Enslaved Healers of Eighteenth-Century Saint-Domingue*. Urbana: University of Illinois Press.

Wendland, Claire. 2010. *A Heart for the Work: Journeys through an African Medical School*. Chicago: University of Chicago Press.

WHO. 2006. *Working Together for Health: The World Health Report 2006*. Accessed August 31, 2009. http://www.who.int/whr/2006/overview/en/index.html.

World Bank. 2007. "Summary of Discussion and Agreements Reached during Technical Meeting on Aid Coordination and Budget Support." Summary Report. Accessed April 5, 2009. http://siteresources.worldbank.org/INTHAITI/Resources/March23Mtgsummary.pdf.

——. 2011. *Haiti: Migration and Remittances Factbook*. Accessed May 16, 2012. http://siteresources.worldbank.org/INTPROSPECTS/Resources/3349341199807908806/Haiti.pdf.

Wubneh, Mulatu. 2003. "Building Capacity in Africa: The Impact of Institutional, Policy and Resource Factors." *African Development Review* 15 (2/3): 165–98.

Index

reciprocity/"giving back", 62–67, 114–116
religion
  Christian saint archetype (*see* saint
    archetype)
  faith-based vs. secular organizations, 14, 47
  missionaries, 74, 75, 79, 155n2
  spiritual- and plant-based healing, 3
  Vodou and magic, 105, 131
  See also Catholic church
remittances from other countries, 79, 93, 94,
  116, 152. *See also* emigration
rescinding/stopping aid, 63–66
residence abroad. *See* emigration
residents at Hôpital Universitaire Justinien, 13,
  14, 71, 78
  access to modern equipment and materials,
    99–100
  "brain drain" emigration, 92–95
  contracts for foreign training in exchange for
    practice in Haiti, 96–99
  demographics, 79
  Dr. Célestin, 1, 2, 70, 91
  education and training, 78, 88, 89, 96–99
  housing, 82, 83
  interviews, 78
  involvement with international
    organizations, 87–89
  mentors, supervisors, and senior colleagues,
    80, 81, 83
  opinions regarding foreign medical workers,
    87–91, 110
  patients' underappreciation, 100–102
  within professional hierarchies, 79
  "real medicine", 99–102
  salaries and compensation, 82–87
  strike protest by, 82–87
  United States Medical Licensing Examination
    (USMLE), 92
rice and flour, 35
Rieff, David, 6
Robbins, Joel, 119
rural areas, 10, 11, 76, 98, 109
  Cuban medical workers, 108
  Estelle (aid worker), 118, 119, 139–141
  mobile clinics, 14, 19, 31, 118
  negative experiences, 81
  unusual pathologies, 19
  See also Farmer, Paul
Rwanda, 122

Sachs, Jeffrey, 120
Sahay, Anjali, 93

saint archetype, 122–133
  charisma, 120, 129, 131
  Haitians, people who identify as, 133
  requirements to achieve saintly status, 133
  villain-champion dichotomy, 146
  villain-saint dichotomy, 127, 146
  whiteness, 144–146
  women as, 132
  See also Farmer, Paul; Schweitzer, Albert
salaries and compensation, 1, 47, 80, 107,
  108, 126
  chèk zonbi (zombie checks), 158n1
  comparison of Haitians' and foreigners'
    salaries, 90
  debtor relationship of Haiti to resident
    medical workers, 114
  emigration for improved salaries, 81, 94, 95
  strike protest, 82–87
sale/resale of donated items, 133
saying no, 33, 34, 62, 112, 115
  begging/solicitation in public places, 29, 30
  villain archetype, 135
scan diagnostic equipment, 94, 99. *See also*
  technologies
scholarships and subsidized training, 96–99
Schweitzer, Albert, 120, 128–131, 133
Scott, James, 104
security guards, 34
self-interest, 107–109, 134
Sierra Leone, 41
skin color
  complexity of racial classification system,
    136, 137
  stratifications, 119
  See also race issues; whiteness
slavery, 113, 123, 136
slogans on T-shirts, 111
social justice ideals, 106
sovereignty, 41
  within debtor/creditor relationship,
    113, 115
  US debtor/creditor relations with Haiti, 113
Spanish language, 22
stealing. *See* theft
sterilization of hospital linens, 44
stipends. *See* salaries and compensation
Street, Alice, 12, 102
strike protest by residents at Hôpital
  Universitaire Justinien, 82–87
structural violence, 123
subsidized medical training, agreements
  stipulating return to Haiti, 96–99

www.ingramcontent.com/pod-product-compliance
Lightning Source LLC
Chambersburg PA
CBHW030332270326
41926CB00010B/1597